Oh, My Health... There IS Hope

(Book 2 in The Hope Book Series)

by Jana Short

Cathy Mckinnon, Christi Davis, Deni Carruth, Dr. Dixie Short, Dr. Tawnie Lowther, Kara Krueger, Kela Robinson Smith, Melanie Pigeon, Merilee Ford, Nicole Buratti, Tricia Collyer, Scott Gates, Sonja Stuetz, Stephanie Lopez Gilmore, Susan Tillery, Tamica Lloyd

ISBN 978-1-7771144-3-5

Dedication

This book is dedicated to my three sisters, Leslie, Lori, and Lisa, as well as my three daughters, Dr. Tawnie, Casey, and Dr. Dee. They have always showed me what it means to be a powerful, inspiring, and compassionate woman. They are what held me together and inspired me to follow my dreams.

To the love of my life, Steve, who reminds me that, when I dare to be more, I become more.

Thank you to my seven beautiful grandchildren who inspire me to stand up and continue to create a ripple of hope throughout the world. They remind me every day how books like this one create change for their futures.

Contents

Introduction

Serena Carcasole

President, Amazing Women Media, Inc.

Dear Reader,

The very first thing I want to say is that there *is* hope.

You *can* heal yourself, and become empowered to live a healthy, vibrant life, and to enjoy all your favorite things and people.

At the moment, it may seem like feeling great again is impossible. Whether you're struggling with a chronic health issue or experienced a traumatic event and the resulting stress is making you sick, you have within you everything you need to heal yourself and rediscover true well-being.

The good news is that health is so much more than the food you eat, the exercises you perform, and the supplements you take.

It's about *all* of you.

Armed with the right information and inspiration, you can master your own fate.

I know because I've done it. The stress, anxiety, and depression I experienced before and after my father's death led to serious health issues that impacted my ability to live a life I loved.

I'm still living with those health issues, but because I've learned how to manage the stress, anxiety, and depression, I'm dealing with them more effectively.

You see, health problems are like weeds … and the stress, anxiety, and depression are their roots. Only once I dealt with the roots could I manage and control my symptoms.

I learned that healing myself from the inside out was the only way to change my life – for the better.

I also realized I wasn't alone; more importantly, I knew I had to spread my message of hope! I created the "Hope Book Series" as part of my mission to create a movement of holistic success for women around the world.

This book is a collection of stories by and about a group of amazing people who faced and overcame obstacles that felt unbeatable.

Their experiences and healing methods and techniques are as unique as they are.

One thing they all have in common is that they took responsibility for their own health, and they took action to heal themselves and create the positive change they sought. They found options that worked best for them, and used them to transform their lives.

These are people who found hope ... and created health.

Jana Short, this book's lead author, is a perfect example of finding hope in the darkest of places. After a long journey during which she became so sick she nearly died, she made a decision: to go beyond living day-to-day and begin creating memories with her family. This decision not only changed her perspective, but it also opened the door to opportunities that ultimately helped her begin to heal.

Jana, along with each contributor in this book, wants to help you begin to heal, too. That's why each contributor shares a complimentary gift designed to guide you in taking action to create positive change in your life, starting now.

Of course, this book isn't meant to replace advice you receive from your doctors and other healthcare providers; it is meant to give you the inspiration, motivation, and above all, the assurance that healing is possible.

As you read through the stories in this book, I know you'll feel yourself begin to relax, to breathe just a little easier, knowing that your fate is in your hands.

There is always hope.
There is always a way.

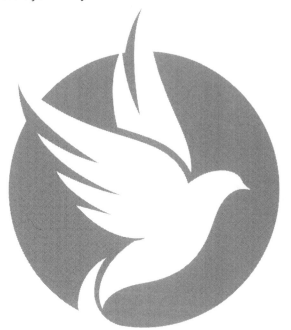

Chapter 1

Living in the Moment, Because the Moment Is All We Have

By Jana Short

About ten years ago, I was required to have a simple fundoplication surgery to fix a small hernia in my esophagus. It should have been super easy. And at first, it seemed to be.

The procedure was completed without a hitch, and I was on my way home the next day. For months, I had no idea anything was even wrong.

Then, I started noticing that, every time I ate, it felt like the food was poisoning me. My stomach would bloat, and I was in constant pain. I of course went back to my doctor and was diagnosed with a bleeding ulcer. Over the next few months, while receiving treatment for the ulcer, my symptoms worsened, and my stomach became so distended, people kept congratulating my husband and me on our pregnancy. (I was actually flattered, seeing as I was getting ready to turn 50!)

The pain intensified, and I ended up in the emergency room. One ultrasound later, the bleeding ulcer ruled out, but a large mass in my stomach was discovered. Several more uncomfortable tests later, the doctors discovered that my previous surgery had damaged my vagus nerve—the tenth cranial nerve (or CN X)—which interfaces with the parasympathetic control of the heart, lungs, and digestive tract, stimulating movement in the latter. My nerve was damaged to the point that nothing I ate was exiting my stomach, and the nutrients my body needed to survive were not being adequately absorbed.

After seeing several experts in the field, doctors decided to treat my condition by removing my stomach. And on April 5th 2012, my entire world changed.

I still remember the car ride to the hospital—me, so naive in thinking what I was about to go through wouldn't alter my life as I knew it.

The surgery itself seemed to go very well. A few days into my recovery, I was able to start taking in Jell-o and other soft foods. Around the fifth day post procedure, I was eating some mashed potatoes, and I remember the nurses suddenly rushing in and snatching away my tray and water container.

The greatest risk of complications from any surgery had occurred—dehiscence. Somewhere inside my stomach, my surgery had opened, and it was pouring out the foods and liquids I had been consuming into my body cavity. Things quickly went downhill from there, and I became septic, with a horrible case of pancreatitis. I became very sick, very fast. I was in fact so ill that going back in for a second surgery was never an option.

I don't remember a whole lot of what went on at the time, but I do remember always thinking ahead, and continually saying to myself, "If I can just get through today, tomorrow will be easier." I spent six weeks in the hospital, struggling to stay focused on that very thought. My husband was the only person I would allow to visit, and he came every single day. I know my recovery was strongly related to the fact that I had him as my advocate during the entire ordeal. He knew how much I hated being there, too, so he even somehow got permission to unhook most of my equipment and put me in a wheelchair daily, so he could take me for a quick ten-minute walk outside in the sunshine.

Even though I refused to let my family visit me in the hospital (the last thing I wanted was for them to see me in that condition, knowing how they would worry), my husband also arranged a surprise for me on my 51st birthday. Wheeling me outside for one of those sunshine recharges, I saw my entire family there on the grass with balloons and flowers. Best medicine EVER! (In retrospect, I regret not allowing them to see me, as I realize it was actually selfish of me. That's a mistake I would never repeat again.)

After six weeks in the ICU, running my mantra ("Just get through, today, and tomorrow will be better,") through my head over and over, I had enough. I broke down crying; I did not want to die in that hospital bed. I begged my doctor to let me go home. I felt as though all the medicine they were pumping into my IV's was draining me of life. He agreed that even though my open wound had not healed, they had done all they could for me, and it would probably be better for me to be home with my family. (This doctor was so amazing that he called me every morning at 7:00 AM for the next two months to check on my wellbeing.)

And that's when the magic started.

By this point, I had not eaten or drunk anything orally for almost two months. I was required to carry a backpack for 18 hours a day that pumped TPN (Total Parenteral Nutrition) into my body that bypasses the digestive system to nourish me. Of course, my body didn't like it, and it was starting to affect my organs. Not only that, but the backpack was so heavy that for the first four hours of the day, I couldn't even stand up while wearing it, let alone have the strength to carry it around.

Now that I was home, I needed to see my family. One of the very first people who came to visit was my daughter, who had just given birth to her second son, our fifth grandchild. He was around six weeks old, and I remember holding him with tears in my eyes. It had dawned on me that he may never have a single memory of me; he might never know how much I adored and loved him. I decided right then and there that, although I might be going sooner than I'd like to, nothing was going to stop me from making memories with my family in the time I had left.

I changed my mantra, and I believe it saved my life. Instead of thinking, "If I can just make it through today, tomorrow will be better," I started repeating this: "Just let me make one more memory to leave with them, and to take with me."

I began a new journey then … one that centered around creating memories with those I love so much. And on that journey, I experienced miracles.

As weak and sick as I was, I decided to take my family to visit our relatives in Utah to create some fantastic new memories. I packed up my backpack, loaded two cars, and we hit the road.

That newborn little grandson of mine had some plans of his own. Like a lot of infants, he was struggling at the time with horrible colic. He was miserable, screaming in discomfort for hours at a time. I felt so terrible for him and watched protectively over him as my cousin offered to rub some lavender oil on his tummy. Within a matter of minutes, I watched his whole body change as the tension seemed to melt away and his entire posture relaxed. I could hardly believe my eyes! I became so curious, immediately asking tons of questions about the oil. What was it exactly? What was in it? How did it do what it just did? And the whole time, in the back of my mind I was shouting *CAN IT HELP ME, TOO?* I was so excited when my cousin said there was a class I could attend the very next day about essential oils.

I admit, I almost walked out of that class! There were a lot of women present who were seeking information about using oils to help their babies with things like diaper rash, teething, and fevers—none of which pertained to me. I was dying and out of time! But I swear the best thing I ever did was wait it out to speak to the amazing woman who hosted the class. She shared knowledge and a sample bottle of oil with me that changed the course of my life.

Using the sample, I started feeling better quickly. Of course, I did what most everyone does, and doubted that it was actually the oil. In my mind, it couldn't have been. No, surely I was just *supposed* to get well. I wasn't supposed to die so soon. I wasn't ready, and my body was just finally starting to heal.

But a couple of weeks later, that sample bottle had run out. I had placed an order but honestly forgot all about it. Just a couple of days without the oils and I relapsed with a vengeance! I was back in bed, weak and sick. My husband, who to this day is not a huge fan of holistic anything, found that small box of oils I had ordered and brought it to me — holding it out to me as a precious offering of hope. Within 24 hours of using my digestive oil, I started improving again.

It has been nine years now, since that trip to Utah that changed everything. I have since gone through 15 surgeries, including a double mastectomy, ovariectomy, multiple reconstructive surgeries, sinus surgery, and vascular surgery. And here's what's crazy: I have never felt stronger! I eat pretty much whatever I like (of course, it sometimes comes with a price). While I didn't miraculously grow a new stomach, and still have tons of issues, I now have the most incredible, manageable quality of life! I love traveling, and I go on a vacation with all my grandkids every summer since the first summer I made it home from the hospital. I ran a two-day, 200-mile RAGNAR relay race with my oldest daughter and younger sister. (I had never run a day in my life before, but trained for six months to complete the three legs of this race.) My husband and I have been able to take several dream trips, to Prague, Peru, Patagonia, and Africa. And best of all, I have been given TIME—time to create more memories with my loved ones.

I live in the moment, now, because the one thing I know is definite is that the moment is all we are sure to have.

Now, it is crucial to me that I make it very clear that I did not *cure* anything with magical bottles of oil. There is no magic pill! But I did experience a transformation that I attribute in part to the oils that I now know can make a huge difference in our health.

My transformation occurred in baby steps. It took a ton of hard work, lots of failed attempts (which were blessings in disguise, as I took something away from all of them), and a commitment to constantly educating myself in a completely different manner than I was used to.

Because of my own experience, I now work as a Holistic Health and Wellness Coach and NLP Practitioner. I have grown a vast online following that has enabled me to extend my reach globally. I started collaborating with other experts in the field of holistic wellness working on books, summits, podcasts, and blogging, to get our stories of hope out there to reach as many people as we possibly can who need them most.

If you are one of those people … if you're at a place in your life where it seems very dark, and you're struggling for answers, I want you to know you are worthy of finding solutions. There IS hope, and you can create an incredible quality of life you deserve.

Jana Short

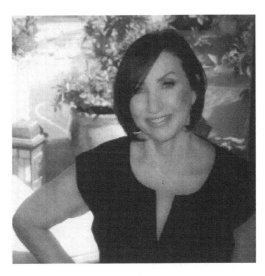

Jana Short is an NLP Practitioner and Wellness Coach, and the founder of Best Holistic Life Editorial Blogging site and Health Influencers Mastermind, connecting real experts and major health influencers who offer their services online with their dream clients. She helps coaches increase their reach globally, thereby allowing them to share their expertise through speaking engagements, book collaborations, podcasts, magazine features, and contribution space in Best Holistic Life editorial blogging site. Jana recently released her Podcast Oh, My Health... There is HOPE! wherein she continues to share stories of hope with her listeners.

To connect and collaborate with Jana, join her on Instagram @bestholisticlife, or read more about her at janashort.com and bestholisticlife.com. You can also tune into her podcast Oh, My Health... There is HOPE!

Get Jana's free gift, **How to Improve Your Self-Care in 30 Days**, here: hopebookseries.com/gifts.

Chapter 2

One Size Does NOT Fit All!

By Dr. Dixie Short

Have you ever noticed just how unique we all are? If you haven't, I challenge you to find two people who are identical in ALL aspects. That would be impossible, right? Even identical twins have differences.

The truth is that we are all different for important reasons. For example, if it weren't for our differences, everyone in the world would be allergic to the same things, have the same reactions to medications, eat all the same foods, wear the same size … the list goes on and on. Plus, consider this: If everyone w the same, what could kill one person could kill everyone.

Now, there are benefits and detriments to genetic variation. One of the greatest benefits is the ability to create antibodies, which is the genetic equivalent to taking someone else's proven defense mechanisms and adding them to *your* current defensive strategy. For most people, it's a game changer. On the flip side, one of the greatest downsides to genetic variation is that we all react differently to everything. Again, in some cases, this works to our advantage. But unfortunately, there are also instances in which it causes a sort of "domino effect" in our lives and overall health. In fact, I have experienced firsthand how inconvenient it can be to fall outside the norm when it comes to medicine.

I have always wanted to be a doctor. When I was four years old, my great grandmother died of a heart attack in my arms. I was so afraid; I had no idea what was wrong with her. At the time, she had said she was not feeling well, so I did what my parents did for me when I was sick. I put a damp washcloth on her forehead and sang to her as I rocked her on the bathroom floor. That's how my parents found me when they came home—with her in my arms, thinking she had simply fallen asleep. It was this incident that created my fierce commitment to never again losing someone I loved due to my own ignorance.

So I started to read anything I could get my hands on that might be of value to me in service of that commitment. My parents still have pictures of me reading medical textbooks in the corner of our living room at the age of five! Needless to say, I ended up with more questions than answers.

Throughout my academic career, I tried my best to jam as many courses and areas of study that into my schedule that I could to give myself the "leg up" in preventing the inevitable. In high school, I was enrolled in a minimum of eight courses at all times, ten clubs, various sports, choir, and additional education off campus. When it came time for college, I got to customize my own education, and I was like a kid in a candy store doing so. I wanted—no, I was *driven*—to learn everything I possibly could. I triple majored in Nursing, Gerontology, and Biochemistry. I was on campus over fifteen hours a day six days a week. And that's when I started to notice a major decline in my health.

Now, to the outside observer, the cause seems relatively clear, right? I was obviously not taking care of myself, and was constantly overworked and overstressed. And that's exactly what multiple doctors told me. Their prescribed "treatment" was to schedule in more downtime. Like most people, I took their advice to heart and implemented their suggested treatment into my life. But I continued to get worse.

I watched my health progressively decline even as I cut way back on my workload, averaging about ten-hour five-day work weeks. I incorporated a number of stress-reduction techniques into my daily life as well, including routine spa nights, meditation, and yoga. Yet despite all these new preventive measures I was taking, I continued to deteriorate to the point of having to take time off from school completely, because I couldn't make it through even one class without having to leave to vomit.

By my thirtieth birthday, I had reached my breaking point. I decided it was time to focus on my health and self-care, and subsequently dedicated an entire year to focusing only on that.

So, on that birthday, I went to the doctor for a compressive physical and routine bloodwork. I waited about two to three hours, and my appointment took about five to ten minutes. My doctor told me that I had a severe sinus infection and prescribed me six different medications. She seemed so confident in her diagnosis, I was truly hopeful that I finally had the reason behind my poor health, and of course, the solution. But the medications didn't work—I still felt terrible. After two weeks, I went back to that doctor. Repeat the same cycle of waiting two to three hours to be seen for five to ten minutes, receiving another six different prescriptions. This same cycle went on for a full year, until I finally decided that there *had* to be another way. Clearly, traditional medicine was not for me. I realized it was time to treat myself like the "unicorn" I clearly was, and I began looking into alternative medicine.

At first, like most people, I was very skeptical. I had been raised to approach my problems by breaking down the things I could see and analyzing them. Everything I had been taught in school engrained that process of reasoning into every aspect of my life. Needless to say, that approach doesn't quite work with alternative medicine.

I tried acupuncture first. The acupuncturist had me rank my pain level prior to the treatment and again after. I went in at a ten and left at a four, and that was it—I was sold! I started to go to that acupuncturist regularly, and during those visits, I told him about my medical issues. He suggested I look into Ayurvedic medicine. Again, I was a little skeptical … until I read about the "tongue-and-nail diagnosis." When I tried it, it told the same story my bloodwork did! The fact that you could diagnose someone in such a simple way absolutely blew me away.

So I started reading up on the foundation of Ayurvedic medicine—nutrition. It made perfect sense to me that what you put into your body determines what you get out of it. In all those years of being sick, my doctors had never once discussed diet and nutrition with me. Despite all the classes and education and books I immersed myself in throughout my life, I had only ever taken one nutritional course. Looking back now, it seems crazy that I had to take so many classes on prescriptions but only one on nutrition!

What I know now is that nutrition is *the most important ingredient* in a healthy lifestyle. Yet we receive little to no information on what our bodies truly need to be healthy, or how to identify a lack of important nutrients.

After incorporating the Ayurvedic nutritional aspect into my daily routine, I saw results within thirty days, and I was blown away by the difference: I was no longer vomiting, my heartburn was gone, I was sleeping, and I was no longer regularly sick. Best of all, I was no longer using ANY prescriptions!

It was at this point that my passion for knowledge was restored, because I knew there were people out there in the same place I had found myself—desperately seeking help. I so wanted to provide them with the solution I had found to help them reach their health (and life) goals. So, with my mother's help, I found and enrolled in a school for natural medicine. I burned through the "work-at-your-own-pace" course work. I loved learning new techniques that I could apply to treat people in a natural, safe, and holistic way. I couldn't graduate soon enough! My own experience taught me that everyone *is* different, and that lasting results do not happen overnight. That's why it's imperative to have as many options as possible for our clients. It also goes a long way in in creating a *customized* healthcare plan specific to the individual ... designed entirely around that one unique individual.

I can honestly say that natural and alternative medicine changed my life. And I have seen it work for *so* many different people. One of my favorite things about it is how practitioners spend so much time (as opposed to the ten to fifteen minutes you often get in a traditional doctor's office) focusing on *all* aspects of an individual's life to identify areas that have been affected by illness. Alternative medicine focuses on treating the patient as a whole rather than just treating or masking the "side effects" that are actually our body's subtle way of letting us know there is a problem.

If you find yourself in a similar situation as mine, or you are looking for a safe and effective alternative to improve your health, I would love to help you on your journey to a healthy and happy lifestyle!

Dr. Dixie Short

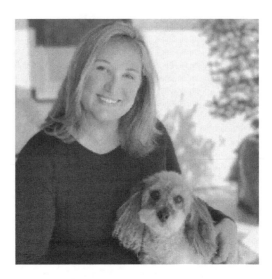

Dr. Dixie Short (aka Dr. Dee) is a DNM, with a PhD in Natural Medicine. She is dedicated to helping people establish healthy habits to create a natural, healthy, joyful way of living. She believes that by focusing on nutrition, we can rebuild our bodies from within. She can be reached at DrDeeandMe@gmail.com. You can also get some quick tips and helpful information here: AskDrDee.com.

Get Dr. Dixie's free gift, **The Importance of Self-Care Workbook**, here: hopebookseries.com/gifts.

Chapter 3

From Rags to Riches—A Story of HOPE

By Tawnie Lowther

My entire world changed when I was just 21 years old.

I was living with the man I loved … the one I was going to marry. My family disapproved of him, but I knew they would come around. After all, he was going to be part of the family soon! I was confident they would grow to love him as much as I did.

But I guess they were right all along, because Mr. Wonderful put me in the hospital.

Afterward, my mother insisted I stay with her in Washington State for recovery. The estate—a mansion on a lake—was picturesque. (It literally took your breath away.) Before I knew it, weeks turned into months. My friends back in California kept sending me letters … "Are you okay? When are you coming home?"

I didn't have the answers. My ex had managed to get the address of where I was staying, and pleaded for my return. My mother was scared; she knew if I went back to him, I would fall back into his spell and get hurt again—maybe even killed. So, I just stayed where I was.

I remember the day that changed everything. I took my shoes off and walked down to the doc, the sand between my toes. Sitting by the lake, I thought about how peaceful it was there, and how calm I felt. I wanted to keep that feeling forever, so I consciously locked it inside me. When I walked back up to the house, my mom (who was her boss' personal assistant and financial advisor) asked if I would stay for a few more months and help manage the house. She said I would support the maid and eventually become one. I decided to give it a go.

During my downtime, I started drawing. And I can't explain why, but what kept coming to me was a fascination with the human body and earth. In fact, it overtook me, and my drawings reflected that. I drew the brain and body parts connecting to the earth all the time. I still have some of them (like the part-tree, part-human lady I drew in 1998). I bought anatomy and physiology coloring books, and lost myself in coloring them at night.

It was over six months later when my temporary position at the mansion came to an end, and it was time to move back to California. All I had to my name was a brand-new car and about 20 bucks in my pocket. So, as soon as I arrived back home, I grabbed the LA times to look for a job. I was lucky; there was an ad for a maid position in BelAir, in which I could utilize my newly found skills learned in Washington. I got the job, and it ended up being a conduit for my transformation. They were amazing people who treated me like family, and it helped me get on my feet. I was making good money, and one day, I decided to treat myself to my first massage at a local day spa. It was terrific, and I loved everything about it!

I knew I didn't want to be a maid forever, so I enrolled in IPSB (Institute of Psycho Structural Balance) to learn massage therapy. But this particular (renowned, although I didn't know it at the time) school wasn't just about massage—it was actually a natural healing school that offered massage training. It also offered courses in Craniosacral Therapy, Polarity, Grounding, Chakra Cleansing, Reflexology, Acupressure, and many more modes of therapy. And they practiced what they preached … saging students before they entered the room to clear negative energy, guiding us in meditation before and after class. The amazing thing for me was that, even though these types of things were foreign to me, I loved them! I felt they belonged to me, and were part of me.

And that's what prompted me to begin researching how to become a natural medicine doctor, which led me to touring a school in Encino, California that also offered acupuncture programs. I knew it right then and there—I was doing it! And I noticed that the feeling I locked inside me that day at the lake was there inside me … it had become a part of me. And I knew that's what I wanted to share with other people. It had become my mission.

The reality was that I couldn't afford to attend that school in Encino. But I decided I wouldn't let that stop me from doing what I love … HEALING. So, two years after finishing massage school, I planted my feet in a Chiropractic office in Rancho Cucamonga as a massage therapist. And I *loved* working with patients! Not only did I get to use my skills as a massage therapist to help people feel better, but I received additional training, learning to use the Tens unit, ultrasound, and traction. I even got to assist in doing some of the X-rays. I eventually also began taking a reflexology class on weekends at IPSB, to continue my education in natural medicine.

The problem was that the school was over an hour away, and the commute began taking its toll. So, when it was time to register for more classes, I didn't.

But I wasn't ready to stop learning. One day, I went to the library and grabbed the book, "Brain Longevity," by Khalsa, Dharma Sing, M.D., and Cameron Stauth. I don't think I picked this book; I think it chose me. Because just like with my drawings, I was pulled toward learning about the human brain. And that's when the greatest door opened for me.

I wanted to go back to school and learn more, and during this time, I met the head of management at a significant sleep center in LA. I immediately took interest in the field of sleep medicine, because studying sleep involves brain activity studies. And they offered me the most amazing opportunity: they would train me for free—I could learn from management and the doctors themselves—until I could apply for the paid position of certified technologist. The only thing they asked of me in return was my promise to take the boards after completing the hours they would be required of me. This was an unpaid position, and the center was over an hour drive from my home.

How could I commit to driving back and forth, and working all night for free?

I knew the answer; I would do it for the amazing opportunity that had been placed in front of me!

So, I did exactly that, for four months. I kept my promise and passed the boards, and they hired me for the position.

After two years, I applied for a sleep position closer to home at Kaiser Sleep Center in Fontana. I was hired as a Lead Scorer, scoring the sleep test and continuing to work the night shift. It was a great experience, and I grew as professional in the field. I said goodbye to Kaiser after almost ten years, and then took a position at Eisenhower Hospital as a Sleep Technologist and Clinical Sleep Educator. During this time, my desire to learn about human behavior peaked, and I ended up taking three years of psychology. I also learned how to do EEGs for seizures and other brain activities that needed reporting. I was a sleep tech by night, and an EEG Tech in ICU by day. I absolutely loved working side by side with doctors, and spending time with patients as I helped them heal!

Approximately a year and a half later, I received a call from my mom. She asked if I was sitting down. "I am now," I whispered. Excitedly, she explained how she had found Quantum University, school of natural medicine, for me to look into, and I immediately checked it out online. I called and spoke to some of the staff at the University, and I was impressed. I enrolled, along with my sister. After completing my education there, I finally realized that my dream of becoming a doctor of natural medicine was becoming my new reality.

Here's the lesson I want to share with you:

I never would have realized my dream if the cards of my life had been played *any* differently.

It took 20 years for my journey to lead me to Quantum University. Even though the seed of that calling was planted in me way back when I was healing at the estate in Washington, I wasn't ready then. Every part of my journey to where I am today was essential. I received the training I needed, step by step, until it all came together for me when I was ready and prepared for it.

Admittedly, some of those steps were struggles I wouldn't wish on anyone. But even those became integral parts of my journey. After all, if I hadn't gone to the estate, I wouldn't have had that moment—the one that changed everything—by the lake.

You just never know when your path will lead you exactly where you are meant to be. So remember that, even when that path is bumpy, you've got to keep moving. This walk through life is a journey of discovery … and every single step could lead you to your dream.

Tawnie Lowther

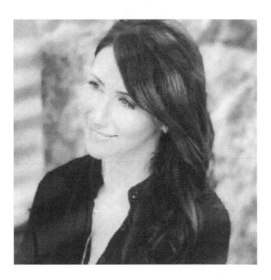

Tawnie L. Lowther, RPSGT, CSE, DNM, PhD, is an accomplished sleep educator, NLP Practitioner and Doctor of Natural Medicine. Having over 19 years of experience in the sleep field, she has dedicated herself to helping people improve their quality of sleep, and thus, their quality of life.

Get Tawnie's free gift—her **Sleep Journal and Tracker— to get one step closer to your health goals by improving your sleep quality**, here: hopebookseries.com/gifts.

Chapter 4

From Homeless to Healthy:
How One Diabetes Coach Is Helping Women Take Their
Lives Back, One Small Change at a Time

By Tamica Lloyd

If you're sick and tired of feeling sick and tired … if your weight or health slows you down, and/or stops you from doing things you enjoy with people you love …

I want you to know there *is* hope.

I'd like you to think for a moment about what will happen if you don't change your health condition. (Go ahead … I'll wait!)

Now, think about what a healthy body looks and feels like. Consider what you'd like your life to be like three years from now. Imagine being your ideal weight, free of medications, laughing, running around with your children or grandchildren.

That feels pretty good, doesn't it?

Here's the good news: no matter where you've been, what you've tried, or where you are now, you can make small changes that lead to big results.

You can get your life back, one small step at a time.

I'm living proof! Not only do I come from a family where many people have Type 2 Diabetes, but I also suffered severe trauma when I was younger. Still, once I made the decision to change my life and improve my health, I did. And now, I'm on a mission to help you do the same.

Here's my story, so you know I understand completely where you might be right now.

Both of my parents died when I was 14. I went to live with a family member, who molested me. Living on the couches of my friends, and on the streets, seemed like the best options at that point.

It was the kindness of strangers—and my own deep, inner knowing that *I was meant for something better*—that ultimately helped me transform my life.

See, I was an angry person. People who had claimed to love me betrayed me, and I felt unloved, unworthy, and ashamed. I felt like God had turned a blind eye.

I began to put on weight. I used food to medicate; subconsciously, I thought that if I was overweight, no one would want me, and I could thereby avoid being hurt.

I knew something had to change. I just didn't know *how*.

During this time, there was a Rabbi who often passed me by. At first, he didn't speak to me, but after a while, he started to ask me about my situation.

I told him my parents were dead and I couldn't live in a home where I was being molested. He advised me about forgiveness—how it would help me heal and keep me sane. He talked about the power I had to ensure my circumstances didn't set my life on a permanent downward trajectory. He introduced me to two books that changed my life: "How to Win Friends and Influence People" by Dale Carnegie, and "Think and Grow Rich" by Napoleon Hill, which talked about the laws of attraction and why people stay stuck in poverty. Both of these books were a godsend!

I began to practice the things I read. I began to visualize having a home where I felt safe and happy—just until I got to college, which was four months away.

One day, I was at a friend's house when my godmother and her friend arrived. When I told them the story of what happened to me, my godmother took me in.

The most amazing thing was that when I actually experienced having that safe, warm, happy home, the feeling was the same as what I'd visualized as part of implementing what I'd read in those two books.

But then, at age 22, I was raped. I took an emotional downward spiral, and it worsened my relationship with food. The more I thought about the traumas in my life, the more I medicated myself with food.

But I never lost the feeling—the belief—that *I was meant for more*. For *better*.

I started to practice forgiveness. I realized I wasn't to blame for what happened to me, and I had to stop hating myself. And things began to change.

As the years passed, I lived a happy life. I became a mom and got married to the man of my dreams. Yet my subconscious continued to try to keep me safe as I used food to soothe myself and ensure I wouldn't be attractive. (The kind of wounds I was dealing with run deep, and my subconscious was still contending with them.)

I weighed more than 220 pounds (which, at 5'4", was OBESE according to the BMI scale).

I was diagnosed with Type 2 Diabetes. My doctor told me to "live with it" and to get used to being on drugs for the rest of my life.

I read enough about the condition to know I *could* heal from it—but I continued self-destructive habits anyway, until, seven years ago, when I ended up in the hospital with Diabetes and anemia.

The first of six weekly iron infusions for my anemia went well, but the second one almost killed me.

One minute I was laughing with my husband … and the next, I was outside of my own body, watching him talk to me, repeating my name, trying to get me to answer him. I couldn't respond.

I watched everything from above … myself, my husband, the nurses running toward me. I tried to speak, but no one could hear me.

I could feel this presence, which I believed was God, and I pleaded for my life. My husband's calm voice, in the distance, talked to my body. I could see the love and fear in his eyes as he kept saying, "Look at me. Don't close your eyes."

I continued to plead with God, promising Him I would make serious changes. The last words I remember saying to Him were, "Please, God, I love you. Please don't take me from my daughter and husband. I promise I will change, and I will help other people if you spare me."

The next thing I knew, I was back in my body, surrounded by doctors and nurses.

I knew God had spared me so I could help other people. So once I recuperated, I kept my promise.

I studied everything I could, like the *China Study* by Dr. T. Colin Campbell, and implemented a whole-foods, plant-based diet. It taught me the power of food, and how what you put into your body has the capacity to harm or heal.

I started exercising—walking five minutes at a time, three times each day. The weight started to drop, and so did my morning glucose level. I gradually increased my walking to a total of an hour each day, incorporated weights twice a week, and the Max Trainer three times each week.

I was experiencing a health transformation, and I just knew I had to share what I had learned. So, I became a Diabetes Coach, to carry out my new mission: ridding the world of Type 2 Diabetes by helping others who have Type 2 Diabetes (or are pre-diabetic) reverse their condition and minimize or eliminate their need for medications.

Along with my training (I'm a Certified Integrative Nutrition Coach), my gifts—healing, listening, and helping people take massive action to change their life—make me an effective coach.

I share my story with you as a form of inspiration. I want you to know that, *no matter where you're standing now (dealing with trauma, addicted to food, unsure of what "healthy" food really is, using food as a reward), if you have a deep desire to get healthy, you CAN, by making small changes that lead to big steps.*

That first step: make one promise to yourself that you can keep.

For me, that was nixing all processed sugars (and those were like crack to me!). Every time I had a craving for sugar, I'd eat a piece of fruit instead. I kid you not; I ate a pound of fruit every day for the first three weeks! Two things changed: I eliminated my cravings for sugar, and my blood glucose levels dropped.

My point is that you absolutely CAN break your food addictions and curb your cravings, and you CAN have a normal life (free from medications, even)—if you're willing to put yourself first and do the work.

All you have to do is take it one moment at a time, one day at a time.

Here are some steps you can start taking immediately to begin your journey to better health—even if you feel like you've tried everything, and nothing has worked:

Step 1. Know you can do it and get positive. Improved health starts with a positive attitude. Even if, like me, you've failed 1,000 times, try for the 1,001st time. I had to "fake it until I made it." You can, too. Read positive stories, read affirmations, do something nice for someone unexpectedly. Kindness lifts your spirits!

Step 2. Juice 16 ounces of organic celery every morning. Drink it on an empty stomach. Most of our health problems start in our gut. Celery juice can heal your digestive tract, lower inflammation, reduce bloating, prevent high blood pressure, help lower cholesterol, protect your liver, curb cravings for sweets, fight infection, and more. (Talk about a "power" food, right?)

Step 3. Eat fruit! Fruits like berries, oranges, kiwi, mangoes, and green apples are beneficial to people with Type 2 Diabetes. Not only do fruits contain antioxidants and fiber, but they also *do not spike your blood sugar*. According to Dr. Michael

Gregor, "Fructose [the natural sugar in fruit] is a dietary mono-saccharide present naturally in fruits and vegetables. Unlike glucose, fructose is NOT an insulin secretagogue [which means the body doesn't use insulin to metabolize fructose found in fruits]. Diabetes is caused by eating too many fats, processed sugars, starches, and bad carbohydrates, and can in fact lower circulating insulin."

Step 4. Eat vegetables, raw and cooked. These foods are full of phytonutrients, minerals, vitamins, and other powerful ingredients that will help your body heal.

Step 5. Eat small meals every two to three hours. Eating small meals more frequently keeps your blood sugar balanced.

Step 6. Exercise. Start small with whatever you can do, even if that's walking 10 minutes each day. Work your way up to an hour each day, or 10,000-15,000 steps.

Step 7. Buy high-quality supplements, including a good multi vitamin, vitamin D, antioxidant, and chromium. (Check out my website at www.isotonix.com/coachtamica for products I recommend.

Step 8. Get at least seven hours of sleep each night. Your body needs time to repair itself, and especially as you go through changes for better health, your body needs adequate sleep to give you the energy you need.

Step 9. Avoid all processed foods, sugars, and fast food. These foods are loaded with chemicals, hidden sugars, and fats that are disastrous to our health.

Step 10. Drink enough water! If you weigh less than 150 pounds, 64 ounces each day is great. If you weigh more than that, drink half your weight in water (so if you're 200 pounds, drink 100 ounces of water each day).

Bonus Step. Keep a journal. Write down at least two things you're grateful for DAILY. The power of gratitude keeps us focused on the good in our life, which in turn brings us more great things.

Your health matters.

You CAN make big changes that lead to a healthy body and healthy mind, simply by making one small change at a time.

Tamica Lloyd

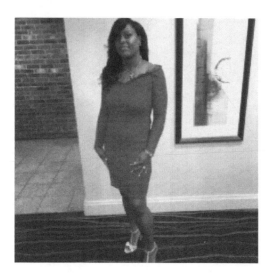

Diabetes Coach Tamica Lloyd is a Certified Health, Wellness, and Nutrition Coach who is passionate about health, fitness, nutrition, and happiness. Her journey began almost a decade ago when she was diagnosed with Type 2 Diabetes and her doctor told her she'd just have to "live with it." That wasn't good enough for Tamica. She started to read everything she could about food and how it affects the body ... and she began to realize she may be able to reverse her Type 2 Diabetes if she changed the way she ate and lived. Within six months, her levels were normal—and she lost 60 pounds. Now, she's on a mission to help other women living with Type 2 Diabetes to heal. You can learn more about her here: coachtamica.com.

To take the first step, sign up for Tamica's free gift, the **5-Day No-Sugar Challenge**, and let her help you curb your sugar cravings: hopebookseries.com/gifts.

Chapter 5

How Mindful Living Can Change Your Life

By Cathy Mckinnon

In our youth, we think we are invincible. Not a care in the world, right?

The moment we actually get serious about life is different for each of us. For some, the universe decides that moment for us. For others, we grow into that moment over a series of events or circumstances.

I didn't see my moment coming. I was living perfectly care-free! That is, before the universe slapped me right in the face with a cancer diagnosis.

The news rocked my world! Up until that point, I never gave any thought as to what I was putting into my body, or how it was impacting my overall health.

The cancer was in my thyroid (the epicenter for metabolism), so it had to be removed. I was also put on a lifelong medication regime, the side effects of which were incredibly overwhelming at first.

At 30 years old, I had no understanding of my own body. It no longer reacted to things the way it used to, and *everything* I had known about diet and exercise had to be revamped! It was like living in a foreign land where you don't speak the language. I had to go back to basics and start all over again.

The deep dive into the hard work began. I wanted to learn everything I could about healthy living, so I researched constantly.

I engrossed myself in learning about healthy living, clean eating, and the endocrine system.

The more I learned, though, the more I realized that everything I knew about nutrition had to be overhauled: it was time to remove dairy and gluten from my diet completely, and become more plant based.

If I'm honest, overhauling my diet was the easier task. Understanding how the food choices you make have lasting impacts on your health is actually an easy-to-understand process.

The more difficult task for me was around the concept of mindfulness.

It was when holistic health came into my learnings that my world truly opened up.

As if changing my entire lifestyle wasn't a big enough undertaking, I soon learned that one of the side effects of the thyroid medication I was prescribed is anxiety. Although I was high functioning, it began impacting my life. I had no idea why no medical professional out of the dozens I had seen ever mentioned it as a common side effect of the medication.

I knew it was up to me—the only person ultimately in charge of my life—to get it under control.

Now, it was also during this time that I also began my journey as a single mom. When my son was with his father, I found myself in an empty, quiet house with a *lot* of time on my hands. I knew I now had time to do things for myself again, but I didn't know what those things would be.

The truth is, I had lost my identity in raising my son. I had to figure out who I was again, and had no clue where to start. I was lonely, I was lost, and I was starting over with a blank slate.

I had to force myself to sit back and gauge what I wanted for my life going forward.

Initially, I started with Yoga classes as a fun way to get out and socialize. However, Yoga quickly became a routine practice I craved weekly as I began learning about mindfulness. I found it so beneficial and I wanted to learn *more*—so I tried out other forms of Yoga and meditation.

I felt better both physically and mentally after my practice. Those around me started to notice changes in me, commenting on how I was showing up differently, lighter, and less stressed. My anxiety was reduced, and I no longer carried anger.

I was living in gratitude!

Here's what I want you to know:

Mindful living—spending time with intention versus going through the motions—in a clear-headed, reduced-stress state *will exponentially improve your life.*

The benefits are incredible: it reduces cortisol (the stress hormone), helps you lose/maintain weight, gain clarity and energy, and live in joy! And all of this allows you to show up in your life as your absolute best YOU.

If you are constantly stressed out and anxious, I'm willing to bet you are also not really present in day-to-day situations.

If you're ready to begin creating the change to live more joyfully now—to live mindfully—here are some of my best tips for doing so:

Step 1: Create clarity around your actions. You owe yourself the time to sit down and write out your vision for your life! So go ahead and grab a pen and paper now, so you can jot down your answers to the following questions:

Where do you want to go?

How do you want to live?

How do you want to feel?

What will that look life?

Keep what you draft here, and as you progress along your healthy journey, revisit it. Check in with how you are doing in keeping to your vision. Reconsider your vision regularly: is it still valid as is? Has it shifted? If so, refresh it, and use it to ensure you are living in alignment with the path you feel called to. Remember, this is your life, and you can change up the vision anytime you want!

Step 2: Dedicate time to yourself for resetting your mind for clarity by utilizing a mindfulness practice. There are so many ways to do this, including guided meditation, yoga, reading, journaling, going for a walk ... your mindfulness activity can be as individual as you!

I also suggest starting small—integrating mindfulness into your daily life does not have to be overwhelming or life altering. Maybe you set aside a certain amount of time each day during which you will turn off all electronics. From there, you can maybe start journaling or reading. Then, you might incorporate a short meditation (think five minutes). (Not sure where to start? Search online for "guided meditations"—there are many online tools to help.) As you gain more practice, you will start to notice preferences. Take note of them, so you can develop your own unique mindfulness habits.

Step 3: Set downtime. The need to be constantly busy is a trauma response to avoid being one with yourself. Allow yourself the time and space to work through thoughts and emotions that simply take up space and weigh on your mind when you ignore them. It can be uncomfortable at first, but doing the hard work and releasing that weight will allow you to move more freely toward the vision you have for your life!

Step 4: Focus on living in gratitude. Let your thoughts revolve around the positive versus the negative. Writing down three things you are grateful for every single day is a simple gratitude practice that easily shifts your mindset into the positive, helping you to stay in joy! Plus, focusing on the present (what you are grateful for now) goes a long way in keeping you from beating yourself up about things in your past and future (i.e., not being where you want to be in your life, etc.).

Step 5: Concentrate on being present. Make a conscious effort to be in the moment, experiencing what is happening in the now, instead of allowing yourself to be sidetracked with other thoughts. Turn your phone to silent, shut out other distractions, and truly focus on the moment in front of you.

If you are struggling right now ... feeling stressed out and anxious and unsure of how to make the changes that could turn it all around ... I want you to know you CAN find the means to manage a new way of living.

My journey with cancer created what felt like an insurmountable task of relearning my body without a thyroid while dealing with the side effects of medication ... but it *became* a manageable task. And in the end, I am much better off!

Remember that to truly understand your health, you have to look at your body, mind, and energy. It's about so much more than diet and exercise; it is also about the thoughts in your mind and the actions they drive.

Your health is the best investment you can make—so why not make it now?

It is time to become to the healthiest, happiest, most inspired version of you!

Cathy McKinnon

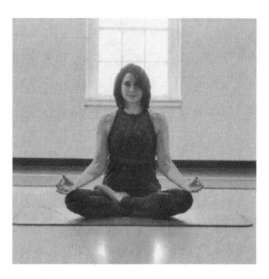

Founder of Wellness Warrior Coaching, Cathy McKinnon works with busy moms to release burnout and FINALLY step into the energy and confidence they dream of … in 90 days! You can learn more about her here: wellnesswarriorcoaching.com.

And be sure to get Cathy's free gift—her **7-Day Self-Love Challenge**—to take matters into your own hands and completely turn your life around in just seven days! Sign up here: hopebookseries.com/gifts.

Chapter 6

Finding Hope: You CAN Stop the Disease Process and Reduce Related Symptoms

By Melanie Pigeon

When is the last time you actually felt *good*? If you can't remember, how angry are you about it, since it likely keeps you from just being you? I get it ... I've been where you are, and let me tell you, it is hard! Thinking back, I was unhealthy for years. I not only struggled with physical symptoms, but with emotional and neurological symptoms, as well. My body was so toxic and sick, it affected every aspect of my being: my ability to work, my identity, my personality, and my relationships. It was a struggle to even be the patient, kind role model I wanted to be for my children ... to be the person I felt good about when I rested my head on my pillow at night. I had wonderful intentions, but there I was fighting myself.

I could remember the person I had been: hard-working, dedicated, reliable, kind, and sweet to her husband. I went to school and earned two bachelor's degrees simultaneously *while* working full time. I met the man of my dreams and landed an amazing job as an ICU nurse. I thought I was doing well—I ate a healthy diet, was at my ideal weight, worked out regularly, and was generally a happy person. Now, I have to be honest: even then, I was no angel, and I'm still not. I have strong opinions, for sure, and bad habits that still come into play today. For example, I tend to stay up late watching smut on TV, which of course makes me moody and symptoms flair the next day. I like to have a drink occasionally, even though I know my body reacts with anger. However, when I am at my best, an occasional treat or late night won't completely derail my healing and stability of symptoms. In the past, that wasn't the case, because I was in a constant state of inflammation.

In reality, I ignored so many symptoms. I remember back when I first became a nurse, I was working in the hospital feeling nauseous, experiencing abdominal pain, and sweating the whole time. I had migraines, rashes, heart palpitations, multiple ovarian cysts rupture (oh, those were fun!). When I ate, it caused bloating and pain. But the symptoms would always pass eventually, and I would move on.

Soon, I developed low blood pressure, and I admit, I chose to view it as a positive: at least I didn't have to worry about high blood pressure! I had seen so many people come into the ICU with uncontrollable high blood pressure, on a handful of medications each with their own set of side effects, and many didn't make it. I also saw what that did to their families, so honestly, I didn't consider my low blood pressure a sign of something bad. So, I continued to ignore the pesky symptoms that bothered me, and just kept moving forward. I got pregnant with my first child, and then my second, and experienced even more health issues. I didn't understand, because again, I thought I was being "healthy"! I ate low fat and whole grain. I "looked" healthy. I remember thinking how unfair it all was, but still, I didn't do anything about it. Then, during my second pregnancy, I began to experience heart-related issues, and almost losing my son at 12 weeks. My doctor put me on bedrest, and my amazing, down-to-earth obstetrician told me I was a "show dog not a breeder," which made me laugh. (Ironically, she and I were both later diagnosed with autoimmune diseases.) I got through the rest of my pregnancy but remained sick throughout the first year of my second child's life. The whole time, I came back to my OB's words, and blamed my body for not being "the breeding type": I was nursing, and my body just didn't like it.

I saw many doctors and specialists and underwent many inconclusive tests before ever getting an accurate diagnosis. With my symptoms, there were many possible culprits on the table, including stress. I'll be honest, that pissed me off! I knew what stress felt like, and what I was experiencing was definitely more than that. Sure, stress was a factor contributing to my symptoms, but it wasn't the sole problem. In my heart, I knew it was likely exacerbating an underlying illness. My lifestyle was stressing my body, creating additional symptoms that I couldn't handle anymore. Looking back now, I realize that my body was trying to warn me—to let me know I wasn't healthy. If only I had listened to it! If I had, I could have avoided getting as sick as I did, ending up with an autoimmune disease that affects my organs. (It's true! I didn't realize it then, but you CAN stop the disease process and reduce related symptoms.)

Here's the thing: When I finally reached the point of desperation to heal, it was because I no longer liked who I was, and I couldn't be an active part of the life I had built for myself (the very one I always wanted!). I had longed to be married and have children. Well, there I was, married with children, and I was too sick, angry, and sad to enjoy it. My husband worked full time, while taking on the roles of father, mother, and caretaker. (Sexy, right?) But I had hit rock bottom, and I was done. I knew I needed to do something other than the mind bashing I put myself through. I knew I was depressed from feeling like I had lost my identity, and that I was headed down a bad path that would likely end with my young boys and loving husband attending my funeral. Doctors told me I wouldn't make it to another decade. And that was my real wake-up call. The problem was, at that point, I had no idea where to turn.

Which is ironic, isn't it? After all, I was a critical care nurse, for God's sake! I kept people alive. I pumped people's chests and brought them back to life. I even educated patients and their families on things like their diet and exercise options when they were released from the hospital. (I know … it's funny!) Yet again and again, I just kept "moving on." (Man, as I write this, it all comes flooding back.) But regardless of all of that, I continued to push and push past it all, until I finally fell.

Hospital visit after hospital visit, I watched my kids' faces at my bedside. Uggg!!! I spent almost all summer in bed, listening to them playing with my husband through the window. Plus, worrying about me caused my husband even more stress than the responsibility he was already carrying as he took over everything and tried to balance it all: the kids, the shopping, his career, the housework. (I'll take the opportunity right now to thank my amazing husband ... thank you, honey! I love you!)

I *had* to figure something else out. I was so sick. I had a newborn and a sick two-year-old who vomited daily, suffered from headaches and constipation, and would become horribly agitated. He was eventually diagnosed with celiac disease—an autoimmune disease. Still, I remained in denial. It's not like that ran in the family, I thought.

Fast forward a few years, when I was finally diagnosed with Lupus, Crohn's disease, and POTS (Postural Orthostatic Tachy-cardia Syndrome). At the same time, my sister was diagnosed with Hashimoto's disease. I started researching, and that's when I first began to understand that health really comes from the inside out. My cardiologist and co-worker in the ICU was a great mentor. He is so knowledgeable about healing from the inside out. He taught me that our gut health is intertwined with our brain health and he had me work on that to control my heart related symptoms as well. He combines western medicine with functional medicine, and it was absolutely life changing for me.

Unfortunately, I will *always* have Lupus, because my body now thinks my heart, vessels, connective tissue, brain, joints, and GI tract (is there anything left??) are all foreign invaders that it must attack. My rock bottom included seizures, joint pain, trouble walking, passing out, fluid around my heart, shortness of breath. and inflammation so bad it affected my brain. There were moments when I couldn't remember anything, or even speak. I remember standing at the sink, wanting to brush my teeth, but not having any idea how to do it. I remember being in a grocery store once, intending to buy bananas, when I just started to cry as I stood there, because I had no idea how to get them.

Eventually, I learned how to keep my system from becoming inflamed in the first place, which keeps my body at rest. And when it is, no attacking occurs. Based on all of this, I created a regimen for others to follow too, so they can stop the attack and heal their bodies.

It requires a commitment to making your health a priority. It's not about medication, but rather a regimen that creates a healthy life. I promise you, no matter where you are right now in your health journey, you CAN stop the progression of your autoimmune disease and prevent the symptoms!

Here are a few tips to get you started:

1. Nutrition:

- Write down *everything* you eat and drink for a full week (don't cheat—this is SO important).

- Cut out all sugar and processed food from your diet (I know, it sounds HARD, right? It gets easier as you go, I swear! The results are rewarding, not restricting, and when you start feeling so much better, it becomes practically effortless!).

2. Sleep:

- Just like we do with our kids, adhere to a set bedtime that allows you a minimum of eight hours of sleep (no, I am not kidding).

- Turn off blue light 20 minutes before bed.

- Write down all the thoughts jumping around in your head (so you effectively put them to bed too!).

3. Tools:

- Take clean, whole-food supplements.

- Add in essential oils.

- Maintain your logs of information, including food, medications, routines, blood pressure, etc.

My goal with this chapter is to help you get to a place of not just feeling "good" again, but the best you have ever felt. The optimal version of you feels restful and comfortable with who you are when you go to sleep at night. That's what I want for you: to learn how to be the healer of your own body, and the sole decision maker for your future, so you can be truly happy.

Melanie Pigeon

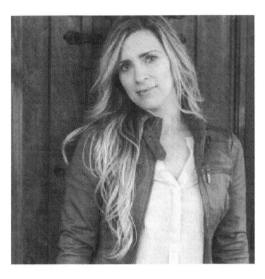

Melanie Pigeon is a nurse and educator, supporting individuals who want to take back control of their health: those who have chronic symptoms and want to discover the cause and solution, and those who have been diagnosed with an autoimmune disease or chronic illness. She is passionate about helping heal those who are suffering, in turn creating happier, healthier families. You can learn more about her here: melaniewellnessrn.org.

And get Melanie's free gift, a one-on-one health consult and personalized nurse care plan, by scheduling it here, right now: hopebookseries.com/gifts.

Chapter 7
Small Changes, Big Shifts

By Patricia Collyer

When you think about health, what immediately comes to mind? If it's "diet and exercise," you're exactly where I was when I started my health journey. After all, that's what we're taught in school, right?

Now, don't get me wrong—both *are* very important in living a healthy lifestyle. But there are many other things that factor into health, too.

Unfortunately, I learned the hard way. The silver lining is that I get to share my story with you now, so hopefully, you can learn from my mistakes instead of by experience.

Not too long ago, I was sitting in my doctor's office for a checkup and mentioned that, along with gaining some weight, I was having trouble sleeping and was irritable more often than I cared to admit. He told me my weight was in the normal range, so not to worry too much, but he'd run some tests to check my thyroid just as a precaution. A week later, my results were in ... everything was normal.

Satisfied with my clean bill of health, I continued with my day-to-day activities as mom, wife, and dedicated employee. My day was pretty typical: get up, get myself and my son ready, make his lunch, take him to school, go to work, come home, have dinner, clean up, stories and bedtime for my son, watch a show with my husband, go to bed, repeat.

I was balancing it all pretty well ... or so I thought.

When my team at work was assigned a big project with a tight deadline, I put in extra time to show my boss my true skill set. At first, it was just a few minutes here and there. But before I knew it, a few minutes turned into an hour or more, and "occasionally" turned into "consistently." I told myself it was only temporary, and justified it with my hope for a promotion (which would benefit my family, too).

However, the extra hours quickly became a point of contention with my husband, so I agreed to leave on time. Still eager to prove myself, I found other ways to put in extra effort. I began eating lunch at my desk and working through breaks, eventually skipping both altogether. To meet deadlines, I took work home at night and on weekends (I was already having trouble sleeping ... why not be productive instead of stare at the bedroom wall, right?).

This worked for a while. And to be honest, I was proud of what I was accomplishing. It felt good to be useful. And that feeling, coupled with my desire to please, pushed me to say "yes" to more additions to the project without adjustments to the already-tight deadline. While I wasn't my happy, optimistic self (I was bottling my emotions as the pressure mounted, and felt like I was spiraling down a dark tunnel practically impossible to climb out of), the feeling of worthiness and pride more than made up for it (or so I told myself, anyway).

Not wanting to lose that new-found pride, I tried my best to hide the fact that I was overwhelmed, exhausted, and burnt out. Struggling to keep everyone happy, I pushed through.

What I failed to see was the true impact of skipping meals, losing sleep, working constantly, and not taking care of myself. I was irritable, impatient, and constantly on edge. I wasn't the mom or wife I wanted to be. I told myself I'd make it up to them, and it would all be worth it once I got that promotion. I thought I could handle the pressure ... until it all fell apart.

I knew I was in over my head; I wanted to ask for help, but I was ashamed. I was afraid it would show my boss I wasn't fit for the job I already had, let alone qualified for a promotion. (I mean, saying "no" at work is career suicide, isn't it?)

Life at home wasn't going well either, but again, I was afraid to admit I couldn't handle it. Everyone else I knew could balance it all. *They* didn't need to ask for help. Who would I be if I admitted I couldn't cut it? I didn't want to find out, so I just kept pretending everything was ok.

But it wasn't.

And one night, it all came crashing down.

Work hadn't gone well that day. First, I was blamed for someone else's mistake and wasn't given a chance to explain. I swallowed my pride and bottled up my frustration. Later that afternoon, we had a project meeting. Every time I spoke, I was interrupted, which kept me from sharing updates and the solution I had found to the major hiccup in our process. Although boiling inside, I managed to keep my cool ... until my boss took me aside on the way out of the meeting and said, "I assumed you would have found a solution by now. I must admit, I thought I could count on you. Now I'm not so sure."

"But I have!" I said.

"Then why keep it to yourself? By not sharing it in the meeting, you're not being a team player," she replied.

"I TRIED!!!!" I barked defensively. Apparently, a little too defensively, because before I could even take a breath, she whipped around and scolded, "Lower your voice; this is an office!" and stormed away.

Mortified, I slumped back to my cubicle desperately fighting back tears.

Drained from work and commuter traffic, I pulled into the driveway. All I wanted to do was melt into my husband's arms and tell him about my horrible day. But instead, I walked into chaos, which was my fault: I was late, which had thrown our entire schedule off. Instead of helping calm things down, I overreacted, trying to explain *why* I was late. I raised my voice. I immediately regretted it and apologized, but the damage was done. The rest of the night was spent in silence ... the house filled with tension.

Once everyone was in bed, I sat in the living room alone and reflected on the day. I started sobbing, all the emotions I had been holding back suddenly crashing down on me all at once.

I *wasn't* the mom I wanted to be. I *wasn't* the wife I wanted to be. I *wasn't* the employee I wanted to be.

And none of it was "like" me at all.

What in the world was wrong with me, I wondered?

If it wasn't my health, what else could it be?

Then, it hit me. (It may be obvious to you at this point, but before that moment, I was clueless.)

I was completely stressed out! I was exhibiting all the signs—overwhelm, burnout, exhaustion, trouble sleeping, negativity, cynicism, irritability, weight gain—and I wasn't taking care of myself.

I was sacrificing myself and my health to please others, and in the process, I was sacrificing my relationships with those most important to me.

Before, I always put "me time" at the bottom of the list. (And let's be honest, here ... who among us consistently gets to the bottom of their list?)

It was that night, when I hit rock bottom, that I realized why they tell you on airplanes to put your oxygen mask on first before helping others. You *have* to take care of yourself in order to be healthy enough to take care of others.

What the doctors never told me was being on constant high alert like I was wreaks havoc on your health! And what I learned on my own is that stress causes the body to react in the same way it would if you were being chased by a lion, tiger, or bear. Oddly enough, that causes a loss of capacity to think creatively, because your blood supply is shifted from your brain to your extremities (so you can run!). Plus, related hormones flood your system causing weight gain and interference with sleep, also thereby depriving your body of the chance to repair and restore balance.

I decided it was time for change. From that moment on, I would reprioritize. My family deserved the BEST of me, not the rest of me. If running myself into the ground was what it took to get promoted, I didn't want it. I wanted to work to live, not live to work! I could finally see how much more important quality of life is than any title or pay raise.

Now, I think about what I want and do my best to align my actions with it. Defining my desires provides a compass, of sorts, that I use to guide my actions. For example, in order to have quality time with my son, I no longer work late. To keep myself healthy—physically and mentally—I drink water throughout the day, bring a healthy lunch, and walk during my breaks.

In order to make those changes, I also had to have some difficult conversations at work. Telling my boss I couldn't work late or take work home anymore, and that I needed my lunch and breaks for myself (not to meet deadlines), wasn't easy. I was even prepared to find a new job if it didn't go well.

It actually turned out to be a very positive experience. Most of my fears were all in my head.

When new tasks or changes to the project came up, I asked what would be taken *off* the list to free up resources to accommodate the change in focus. And you know what? My boss even mentioned how holding boundaries for the project and respecting the time of those involved showed great leadership!

Just by making these small changes, I felt a huge difference in my mood and happiness level. And by taking care of myself, I actually made a positive impact on those around me, as well.

So, what small changes can YOU make, to alleviate stress? Here are some ideas:

Journaling: Writing helps you process your thoughts and feelings, gain perspective, and brainstorm solutions.

Define Your Values and Set Goals: It might seem counter-intuitive, but setting goals helps you define a clear vision of what YOU want, rather than what people expect of you.

Identify Boundaries: Decide what is negotiable and what is not, and stick to it.

Give Yourself Permission to Say No: Consider how requests made of you align with your goals. If they don't fit, say no.

Practice Mindful Eating: Eat when you are actually hungry (as opposed to stress eating), stop when you're full, and be aware of what you are eating (think whole foods versus junk food).

Incorporate Movement: Take a walk! Even if it's just around the office, get moving. Doing so helps take your mind off of whatever is weighing you down.

Breathe: Taking a few deep breaths (watch your belly rise) activates the vagus nerve and tells your body that there is no threat, so it's ok to calm down.

Practice Self-Care: Take time for yourself. Rest. Recharge. It's *not* selfish. You deserve to be at 100%.

Ask for Help: No one does it alone. Asking for help is not shameful or tied to your worth—it shows you care enough to utilize every resource available to be successful.

Trust me, small changes like these can truly shift your entire world—so take it one step at a time, and watch how your life changes.

Patricia Collyer

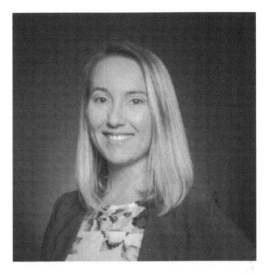

As a certified coach, Trish Collyer's passion is to positively impact the world by helping people create their BEST life. With a background in health, nutrition, personal growth, and communication, Trish strives to support her clients in stepping into greatness as they take back control in their life, so they can achieve everything they desire and more. You can learn more about her here: trishcollyer.com.

Ready to get started? Get Trish's gift to you—a downloadable journal complete with prompts for implementing stress relieving habits—here: hopebookseries.com/gifts.

Chapter 8

From Stress to Success

By Sonja Stuetz

Working in the architecture and building industry for over 15 years, I know a thing or two about stress!

Starting out as a young professional, I wasn't very confident. My lack of experience made me insecure, and the daily demands and pressures quickly became overwhelming. Convinced I wasn't "good enough" to do the job, I worked extra hard and put in very long hours to make up for it—and to prove myself.

As work became my number one priority, it consumed all my time, and I developed very unhealthy habits. For example, I used to be very active, but once the work obsession kicked in, exercise was the first thing that had to go due to time constraints. Then, as workdays became longer, cooking healthy food fell off my list of priorities, too. Regular mealtimes became a luxury, and unhealthy snacks on the go my "nutrition regime." In short, self-care didn't exist for me anymore.

I became obsessed with proving myself. No matter how exhausted and anxious I was, I pushed myself even harder. I told myself that once I had my career "all sorted out," everything would go back to normal. I fooled myself into believing the stress was short term.

Years went by, and I put more and more pressure on myself to reach my career goals. Stress became my "norm" … my way of life.

At first, my body coped quite well with all the pressure (after all, I was young!). And whilst I eventually became more confident and successful in my job, over time, I started to experience various symptoms like sleeplessness, anxiety, and panic attacks. I ignored them all for a very long time.

But then, frustration kicked in. I was unhappy with the way I looked and felt. Poor nutrition and lack of exercise started taking their toll on my body, and naturally, added even more stress.

My loved ones often approached me about working "too hard," but I didn't listen. Even worse, I failed to listen to my own body, which was trying to tell me exactly what I had to do: stop the stressful lifestyle and find a healthy work-life balance.

I learned about the consequences of long-term stress the hard way as I ignored my body's warning signs. Even when the panic attacks and anxiety completely overwhelmed me, I'd stop just long enough to recharge. After a few hours or so, I'd have enough energy to start again, thereby repeating the same toxic stress cycle again and again.

The thing is, you can't recharge an empty battery to 20% and expect it to run like it's at 100% (makes sense, right?).

So, one morning I woke up with my heart racing. I was completely burnt out, and if I'm being honest, scared to death that I had done too much damage to my body to ever recover. It was so bad, I was incapacitated and forced to take a break from my career. My unhealthy lifestyle had finally taken its toll on my health and wellbeing, physically and mentally. I was exhausted, had trouble concentrating, and my body was in pain.

I went to the doctor, and blood tests confirmed my unhealthy lifestyle: I had developed a chronic autoimmune disease.

I remember being so full of questions:

What had I been thinking? How could I treat myself like that? Why was I destroying the wonderful, healthy life I had been given?

Terrified, I started researching stress and coping strategies.

As you are probably aware, stress is our body's natural response to daily demands and pressures. In fact, stress is actually a healthy reaction to challenges, intended to help us cope. As we complete difficult tasks or deal with unpleasant situations, stress can be helpful in that it makes us more alert and energized. Stress is part of life, in that respect, and isolated episodes of temporary stress are usually nothing to worry about.

However, too much stress, especially when experienced over an extended period of time, can affect our health, relationships, work, and general wellbeing in a very negative way.

In fact, when stress becomes a habit, the impact on your health and life can be devastating!

Now, we all know how easy it is to stress—it can be triggered by so many things:

- Work / study pressure
- Job loss
- Insecurity
- Financial problems
- Relationship problems
- Unhealthy diet
- Illness, etc.

And we know stress can negatively affect our emotions, thoughts, and behavior. Right?

But how do you know if things are getting out of hand?

Well, first, you ask yourself the following questions, to acknowledge the existence of stress in your life and to identify what exactly is causing it:

Is my ordinary day ruled by exhaustion, anxiety, overwhelm?

Is my career taking all my energy?

Have I stopped doing things I love in order to free up time for things I don't?

Do I feel like my life revolves around stress?

Do I have underlying health issues, like an autoimmune disease?

Am I experiencing physical symptoms?

Do simple, "normal" tasks feel overwhelming?

If you just answered "yes" to any of those questions, you may want to watch out for the following warning signs:

- Sleeplessness
- Feeling overwhelmed
- Feeling anxious / nervous
- Moodiness
- Lack of motivation / concentration
- Not coping with daily tasks / responsibilities
- Headaches / body aches
- Fatigue
- Panic attacks
- Changed eating habits / weight problems

As I was exhibiting a LOT of these symptoms, I knew it was time for a change.

And thanks to my research, I created that change!

When I started to understand what stress *really* is, I was able to comprehend and recognize what triggers it—the "stress-ors." For example, I became aware of the signs of overwhelm which allowed me to "take charge" of the situation/source of the stress *before* it got out of control … and *that* is what stress management is all about!

I learned how to listen to my body's needs, and implemented various techniques into my daily routine to manage insecurities, workloads, and diet, just to name a few. I slowly developed a system that suited my needs, which ultimately led to a healthy and balanced lifestyle.

One of the biggest keys to my own stress management was realizing that I had choices—I was not just at the mercy of stress beyond my control. And surprise! Everything became so much easier!

Within one year's time, I turned my life (and health) com-pletely around.

Guess what else? Utilizing the strategies I discovered had an unexpected "bonus" side effect: I started to experience more success in my career than ever before!

I began feeling good again, and over time, I even managed to fight my autoimmune disease *without medication*.

Over the last several years, I have deepened my knowledge in stress management, nutrition, physiology, and psychology. I then started a second career as a Health and Life Coach to help others discover how a healthy balanced lifestyle can lead to a more satisfied and successful life.

Here's what I want you to know:

So often, everything seems to happen all at once. Right?

With endless opportunities and information overload, our lives have become more demanding and hectic than ever before.

We will never be able to get rid of stress completely, and really, we shouldn't! As I mentioned before, it can be a helpful reaction to cope with daily demands. However, life doesn't have to be so stressful that it negatively impacts your health! And if you don't listen to your body, it *will* eventually make you listen.

That's why it is so important to learn how to appropriately respond to stressors. You become more resilient, thereby improving your overall health and wellbeing.

Here are three tips for "emergency stress relief on the go" that I've used myself to help me calm down in just a couple of minutes (I hope they will help you, too!).

Tip 1: Take some deep breaths.

When we feel overwhelmed, stressed, or anxious, we often breathe differently, which creates a sort of domino effect on how we feel physically and /or mentally.

Taking a few deep breaths can help you slow your breathing and heart rate, relax your muscles, and calm your mind.

Tip 2: Visualize a place where you felt calm and relaxed in the past.

Imagine yourself in that place, feeling happy, safe, and relaxed.

Whether it was at the beach, on the top of a mountain, or somewhere with someone special ... wherever it was ...

Close your eyes and visualize being there right now. Bring back the memory of how calm and relaxed you felt at that time Remember what you heard, smelled, tasted, and how your body felt.

Now, bring that feeling back to the present moment. Try to relax your face and let go of any tension in your body.

Tip 3: Call someone you trust.

If nothing seems to help you calm down, call someone you trust, like your mum, partner, or a friend. Talk to someone to get your mind off things—doing so helps release negative feelings. Sometimes, just talking about random things will do the trick.

And of course, if you feel like you can't cope, talk to your general practitioner or call a local helpline.

My own journey taught me that, without optimal health, life is compromised in *all* areas.

My hope for you is that you learn how to manage your stress before serious health issues develop.

Believe me, you *can* achieve your goals without sacrificing your health and wellbeing. Even better, once you learn how to manage your stress, you'll be even *more* successful!

Ultimately, you'll increase your chances of living a long, healthy, happy life, as the absolute BEST version of you!

Sonja Stuetz, founder of DIY.systems, is a certified Health and Life Coach. She specializes in a customized systems approach that turns toxic, stressful lifestyles into optimal health. By developing strategies to guide you from stress to success, Sonja's mission is to help you find your ideal work-life balance.

Sonja Stuetz

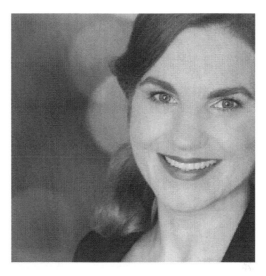

In her spare time, Sonja enjoys traveling, photography, art, and spending time with her family and friends. She also loves to read and play the piano. You can learn more about her here: diy.systems.

Get Sonja's free gift, a one-hour "**From Stress to Success Discovery Session**" (via voice or video chat) to assist you in finding a way out of your stressful lifestyle! Get started here: hopebookseries.com/gifts.

Chapter 9

Why Self-Care Matters Even (and Especially) When You Care for Others

By Susan Tiffery

I've always prided myself on my inclination and ability to take care of others. I believe our influence on others defines how well we've lived.

I chose a career in education for this reason. Over the course of 35 years, I worked in multiple schools and districts, winning Educator of the Year several times. I created and facilitated numerous successful programs, many of which I funded with grants I'd written.

I attribute my success to my passion; I viewed it as an opportunity to take care of people. The downside, though, is that I prioritized my career—and the people related to it—over my own well-being.

From the outside, everything looked fantastic, sure.

On the inside, though, I was burned out and on the brink of collapse. I suffered from brain fog, fatigue, chronic inflammation, and chronic respiratory infections. Needless to say, I was completely worn down. The worst thing: I didn't even realize my symptoms were a result of chronic stress.

I retired early, which should have been an opportunity to change things—to focus on and take care of myself.

But in looking back, I see now that other than stepping away from that busy work schedule, my habits didn't change.

Even though I had more free time, I still didn't prioritize myself or my health. I continued to eat unhealthy food. I didn't exercise. I still felt stressed, and I didn't seek ways to deal with it.

That's when I experienced my wake-up call.

One fall, I went on my dream trip with my family to the mountains above Durango, Colorado. Finding time to take a break from the hustle and grind—especially with my family—was something I didn't take for granted.

During our vacation, we scheduled a guided horseback ride. We had all been riding our entire lives, so I was very comfortable with riding horses, and was really looking forward to it.

The morning of the ride dawned gorgeous, showing off the changing leaves. We left early and headed out onto the trails of the San Juan National Forest.

Just as I swung my leg up and over the saddle, I heard a snap. The instant, sharp pain in my ankle was unbearable. Even Cesar, my equine partner for the day, turned his large nose back toward me, a quizzical look in his eyes.

Determined not to ruin the trip for my family, I settled myself quickly into the saddle. I rode for the next four hours with a dislocated ankle. By the time we returned to base camp and I dismounted, I was unable to place any weight on my swollen ankle without intense pain. I knew then that I wouldn't be doing any more fun family activities for the rest of the trip.

My 84-year-old parents had stayed at the lodge during the horseback ride, and for the rest of the vacation, I stayed there, too. Instead of taking care of them (as it should have been), they had to take care of me. Losing some of my independence and being forced to rely on others was not something I felt comfortable with (*I* am the nurturer, remember!).

The silver lining: the injury forced me to slow down and reflect ... not only on how I'd gotten to that point, but also on how out of alignment my habits had become with how I really wanted to live my life.

Although I'd once played college basketball on a scholarship, and earned my degrees in science, health, and physical education, I was in terrible shape and 50 pounds overweight. I'd spent my entire career teaching other people how to live healthy lives, but I'd neglected implementing my own lessons on health and wellness and therefore, destroyed my own health!

The main culprit? Burnout (the simplest definition of which is "severe chronic stress," and is recognized as a legitimate medical disorder by much of mainstream medicine). While our bodies can handle short-term stress well enough, long-term stress can interfere with normal body functions, such as sleep, digestion, and the immune system. And when these things are out of balance, our mental health suffers.

Science shows that the symptoms of burnout often mirror the symptoms of depression: extreme fatigue, loss of passion, and negativity. Other symptoms include weight gain, anxiety, drops in productivity, and forgetfulness.

That describes exactly what was going on with me. I'd gained weight, I was completely fatigued, and unhappy!

The important thing to know is that this is a *lifestyle-related* condition. In other words, a change in lifestyle can help decrease and heal symptoms caused by burnout.

I believe that the dislocation of my ankle was my body's way of signaling that things had to change.

It was time to focus on my health.

As soon as I returned home from that family vacation, I pulled out the six months' worth of health supplements my friend Amy had recommended to me, that I'd never taken: a combination called "the Triplex," made by a company called Plexus.

Originally, I bought them as an "Ambassador," which meant I got them at wholesale. I didn't realize at the time that my $35 annual Ambassador fee would send me on an amazing journey!

Within just three days of starting to take the Triplex, I was amazed. I went from low energy and craving sugar to high energy and craving water! I felt *great*. The more I learned, the more determined I became to make whatever changes were necessary to get me back to the fully healthy, vibrant, and independent person I once was.

My curiosity had also been piqued: *why* did these supplements work? What was the science behind them? As I researched, my friends and family members began noticing the changes in me. Their curiosity was piqued, too: they wanted what I had—energy, vitality, health ... happiness! They started asking me to get them the supplements, and they, too, experienced incredible results.

Still, even as we were all seeing dramatic improvements in our health and happiness, something was missing: we needed more information about what we should eat, and many of us struggled with things like sugar and coffee addiction. The supplements were a great tool to get us started, but we needed something that would help us make lasting lifestyle changes. It had taken me years to get to the point where I was, and I knew that in addition to the new knowledge I'd cultivated, I'd also need support and accountability to undo the habits I'd gotten into—and more importantly, to create new, healthier ones.

I began to research the science of habit change.

I found Health Coach Institute, an established international coaching certification program. It promised to pioneer the new generation of health coaches who will change the consciousness of the planet.

The Health Coach Institute's curriculum is based on cutting-edge psychology, brain science, intuitive listening, habit change, and healthy lifestyle design, and going through it was truly a life-changing experience. As my physical health improved as a result of what I was learning, I was amazed at how much my mental and emotional health improved, too. It felt so good to be healthy AND happy once again!

All I wanted to do was share what I'd learned with others so they, too, could experience the kind of renewed health, vibrancy, and happiness I was experiencing! (Yes, I'm still a nurturer!)

Finally, I felt like I had all the pieces. When I combined my Plexus health supplements with my new understanding of habit change, I knew I had something truly special to share with others ... something that would transform lives!

That's why I launched my business, Level Up Health and Wellness. In many ways, being a health coach is so similar to what I've done my entire career as an educator, which is to influence others through education. But what is so unique about health coaching is that a coach's main job is to help his or her clients not only learn about themselves but also to realize the profound importance of self-care through the thoughts they have, the foods they choose to fuel their body, the amount of rest they give themselves, and all the things they do (or don't do) for themselves.

Now, I walk the talk. I prioritize and embrace my self-care—the absolute BEST form of healthcare—making it part of my everyday life. In addition to taking my supplements consistently and making healthy food choices, I focus on daily gratitude journaling and meditation. I spend quality time in nature. I listen to uplifting podcasts.

I have shifted my entire mindset!

You may be seeing yourself in this story—you may be on the brink of burnout or deep into it! If so, you *know* you need to get your own health, weight, energy, and life on track. Right? Yet you might also feel like it's counterintuitive to focus on *you* when you feel driven to help others.

I want you to know that in order to help others, *you must first take care of yourself.* When you do, you'll be better equipped to do everything you dreamed of in terms of taking care of your friends, family members, clients, or, like me, students. And if you don't, you simply won't be operating from the best version of yourself—you'll continue to feel drained, exhausted, and depressed.

The truth is, self-care boosts productivity, creativity, and mental health—all of which play a huge role in your ability to care for others (in whatever form that takes for you). Despite the fact that society dictates how we should constantly be busy, working harder and striving to do more and be better all the time, there is no doubt that such a lifestyle is detrimental to our health.

So, here are some questions to ask yourself to determine whether your habits are affecting your health (answer these questions without self-judgment, but with curiosity):

- How do you start your day? Do you practice an attitude of gratitude, or meditate, or do breathing and stretching exercises? Or do you immediately reach for your phone and start checking work emails?

- Do you seek positive, meaningful interactions with other people? Humans are wired to be part of a community, so interacting with those beyond our nuclear family is a big stress reducer.

- Do you have a variety of self-care practices to choose from that require varying time commitments (for example, a few 10-minute practices, a few 30-minute practices, and some that take longer)? How could you fit them in between calls, emailing, and other business tasks?

- How can you fit a little "me" time into each day, around all your responsibilities?

- Do you confuse self-care with self-indulgence? For example, do you convince yourself you deserve that candy bar because you've worked so hard today?

- Do you consistently take health supplements to support your health? (If your response here is, "What supplements?" then we need to talk!)

- Do you regularly get enough sleep?

Why wait any longer to take charge of your health?

The first step: make the decision to take care of yourself—to nurture your body, your mind, and your spirit, so you're functioning from a whole, healthy place. You ARE worth it.

Remember, when you take care of yourself, physically, mentally, and emotionally, you're better able to use your passion to nurture others and change the world.

Susan Tillery

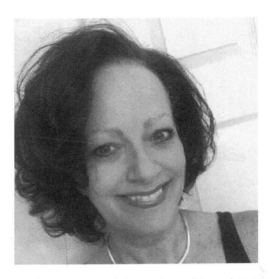

Susan Tillery, the CEO and Founder of Level Up Health and Wellness, has a Master of Science in Education degree and is a Certified Health and Life Coach. With more than 30 years of experience in teaching biology, health, and fitness education, she has curated a plethora of resources and tools to help you get to your next level on your health journey. You can learn more about her transformative programs and life-changing retreats here: levieluphealthandwellness.com.

Download Susan's gift to you—her Self-Care: Your Business's Secret Weapon eBook here: hopebookseries.com/gifts.

Chapter 10

Gramma Judy's Last Gift

By Scott Gates

My In my little town, I have lots of "extended family"—people who aren't related to me by blood, but who are so important to me, they *became* family ... cousins, aunts, uncles, moms, grammas ... who I've essentially adopted. Now, this can get confusing to some (just ask my wife!), but I have been blessed in so many ways by people I consider closer than friends. They are family.

And that's how it was with Gramma Judy—from the moment I met her, she was MY Gramma Judy. The same goes for Jana Short, who I met back in 2012. She became "Mom" so quickly, I can't even remember a time when I called her by her first name. Now, don't get me wrong—I have the most amazing Momma, and no one will ever take her place. But Mom ... well, she has always been so much more than a friend and mentor.

Mom introduced me to the world of essential oils through dōTERRA, and because of that, I experienced a complete transformation in my health. I actually use the term "miracle" to describe it. It's how I began my new wellness path. So, by the spring of 2013, Mom was meeting with me and my friends to help me share with them the many benefits of essential oils, and how they could help them, too. That was so important to me—helping people feel better is the greatest feeling in the world. It is quantum leaps above any satisfaction I have ever enjoyed while previously running my successful IT company. And sometimes, my ever-supportive Gramma Judy would come to those meetings.

It was the summer of 2013 when Gramma Judy and her daughter Darci took a trip to Europe for a month. When they returned, my world was rocked.

They both were so drained. I mean, beat down, as if they'd gone through the wringer. Gramma took naps all the time, all day long, and was always asleep when I went by to see her. She didn't even have the energy to go to the stables with her granddaughter, Tate, to ride the horses, which was one of their favorite things to do together.

A month passed like this. I was at a loss; I so badly wanted to figure out what was happening with Gramma Judy. So, when the next class I had scheduled with Mom approached, I begged the whole family to come. Mom was bringing a new scanner, and I was very hopeful that we could maybe use it to help Gramma Judy. I explained how simple it was to use—you simply hold it in your hand, and working on galvanic skin response, the iTovi scanner allows the body to tell us what oils it needs/wants after just a few minutes. Now, the reason this is so incredible is because, even though I can name over 20 oils can that can help you with say, digestive challenges (or any number of things), no one, not even doctors, can say exactly which one YOUR body will benefit most from. But your body knows, and the scans are basically the medium the body uses to tell us.

You see, everything in nature vibrates at a very specific frequency, and just like a radio, you can tune in to those vibrations. Think of the scanner as a translator—through it, we can ask your body specific questions about what it needs. For example, we can ask it if it needs ginger for the stomach. The body then responds to the frequency of ginger, and algorithms read that response and translates it into a report we can read.

Now, the reports are generated with the oils ranked according to how much the body needs it at that exact moment. It does not tell us why the body needs it. That's why reading the report is a sort of art form, and experience plays a big role in how the report is read.

You see, essential oils support the body in two ways: physically and emotionally. The body may want the oil for one or the other, or both. The report provides a score between 1 and 70: the lower the number, the better. Understand, this isn't like say, cholesterol—a high number doesn't mean you're unhealthy. It simply means your body wants a lot of help from that specific essential oils at that exact moment. In addition, each oil listed also gets a number, which gives us a percentage to help us understand their importance. So, normally we see seven to ten oils on a report, and we focus on the top three. For example, let's say we get a report like this: 60: Deep Blue 22, Wintergreen 17, Cedar Wood 8, Lavender 4, etc. Well, that means that 35% of your score is Deep Blue, and we would then use our experience, a person's answers to our questions, and reference materials to figure out *why* you need Deep Blue.

So, my family walked through the door of that meeting, and after exchanging our customary hugs, I introduced those who hadn't met Jana yet as "Mom." They were all hoping we could scan Gramma Judy before class started, so they could get her back home before she got too tired. "Oh my gosh, of course we can," Mom compassionately replied.

While scanning Gramma Judy, it was like time stood still. It felt like the report took forever to finish. While it was going, we couldn't help ourselves: Mom and I brainstormed the oils we thought would most benefit her. Citrus oils for energy. The immune system blend. The metabolic blend to give her a jump-start.

Finally, we got the score: 38: 36 for Basil and 2 for Wild Orange. Wait, what? Rarely had we ever seen a report come back with only one to two oils listed. Mom and I looked at each other. It couldn't be right. We immediately dug into our books. I grabbed the one based on emotional needs, and flipped to the page on Basil. I handed it over to Gramma Judy to read, and Darci leaned over to read it with her. "Does anything in here sound like what you're going through?" I asked Gramma and Darci. Quickly, they looked at each other, and said, "No, not really." Dejectedly, I took the book back, the feeling of failure welling up inside me.

Mom looked across the table and said, "Judy, can I ask you a personal question, in front of the kids?" I felt my face blush.

"Of course, Jana, shoot." "Have you ever had ovarian cysts, or ovarian cancer?" In my head, I'm instantly thinking, *no way. I would know*.

But Darci sat up and stared. Tate's shoulders slumped in sadness. When I turned to Gramma Judy, I saw it in her sweet blue eyes. I knew it was true.

It was Mom's tapping on my shoulder that brought me back from my daze.

"You've still got Basil in your kit, right?" she asked. As I went to hand it to her, I said to my Gramma, "Please, Gramma Judy, take it. I don't know what to do." Mom kindly stepped in and explained how to use the oil, answering as many of their questions as she could.

They left before class even started. I was humbled by their coming, but couldn't help but feel devastated. Even worse, I felt helpless and wished I could do more.

The next day at lunch, Gramma Judy called thanking me again for the Basil oil. She was following Mom's suggestions for using it, and thanked me for trying to help. She said she was feeling better, and I remember thinking how Gramma Judy that really was ... always supportive of whatever we were doing, so nice, and trying to make *me* feel better.

The day after that phone call, my world was rocked again. She called me back, saying, "Hi, it's Gramma Judy. We need to talk, and you should probably sit down." A lump swelled in my throat. *Oh no*, I thought. *Here it comes*. I imagined I was about to be ostracized from the family for being some kind of "snake oil salesman." "Ok, I'm sitting down," I sheepishly replied.

"I haven't napped at all today, and I even got to go pet Carmel!" "Wait, what? REALLY?!" I exclaimed, beside myself with happiness and relief.

One week later, Gramma Judy rode Carmel, her horse, alongside her granddaughter on her favorite trail, for the first time in ten months. That was the moment that changed my life forever, as I couldn't believe the accuracy of the scan and report.

Three weeks later, I sold my IT company, and began my journey into the world of health and wellness first as an essential oils expert, and soon after, as a Neuro Linguistics Programming (NLP) coach.

Eight months and eleven days after Gramma Judy's ride, Tate called me and said, "Gramma Judy wants to see you now." I dropped everything and went straight home. Because our home wouldn't be "home" without her, Gramma never went to hospice. She stayed with us, her bed in the front room that always smelled of wild oranges, facing the backyard where she loved to sit and read. When I walked through the door (which, in retrospect, probably should have been revolving, considering the number of visitors she always had), she smiled. I was covered in dirt and dust from volunteering at Habitat for Humanity, and she playfully scowled at me as she spoke in her frail, soft voice … "Where do those boots belong?" I'm quite sure I must have looked like a kid with his hand in the cookie jar, as I quietly walked back outside and left my boots at the door, slapping some of the dirt and dust from my clothing.

Returning to her bedside, she looked up at me and clutched my hand in hers. In a soft, now frail voice, she said, "I want you to know what I know." I thought she was about to repeat one of her favorite sayings, which I had heard before: "I want you to know what I know. What you do with it, well, that's on you."

But this time, the words were a little different.

"I want you to know what I know. I know that without you and Jana, I wouldn't have had my last great ride. You gave me the greatest gift I've ever hoped for: time. Because of what you shared with me, I've left nothing unsaid, and was able to comfort those who will need it the most. I have the closure I was praying for. I want you to know that the quality of my life was beyond my wildest dreams, because you shared what you know with me. Don't stop because of me. You didn't fail. I want you to share what you know. If you don't, it's on you."

That was the last time I ever saw Gramma Judy's sweet blue eyes. A week later, she rode on ahead.

It is those last words to me that have become the cornerstone for Gates Wellness.

Now, I'm not sharing this story to suggest that there is a magic oil to "fix" your health. That doesn't exist. What I am saying is that our bodies are constantly trying to heal. It's what they do. And it is my experience that essential oils can assist that process.

Scott Gates

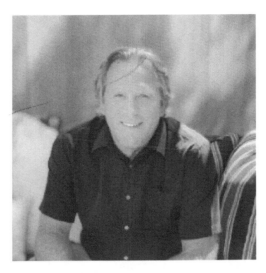

Scott Gates is a Certified NLP (Neuro-Linguistics Programming) Practitioner and Coach, sought after speaker, educator, author, and co-founder of Gates Wellness. In 2020, Gates Wellness will be expanding into the online world of social media and podcasting, and be an ongoing part of Jana's Best Holistic Life and Health Influencers Mastermind Programs. You can learn more about him here: gateswellness.com.

Get Scott's free gift—his **How to Improve Your Self-Care in 30 Days!** eBook—here: hopebookseries.com/gifts.

Chapter 11

Hormones: It's NOT 'All in Your Head'!

By Nicole Buratti

I experienced my "wake-up call" when Kate Spade committed suicide at age 55. Speculation in the Perimenopause groups I'm in on social media brought wonder to the possibility that it was Kate's hormones that drove her to end her life. And the truth is, my groupmates and I could relate to wanting to die rather than deal with what's in front of us.

You see ... I wasn't always the *healthy me* I am now. I worked myself to the bone, eventually leading to burnout in my career, my marriage, and my body. I was hooked on the "coffee-and-wine diet." I let exercise go. As a doula, I pulled all-nighters all the time, and was constantly on call and hyper alert—tied to my phone and Facebook. I ate and slept when I found time to.

Up until age 35, I held my own. I even still got carded when purchasing alcohol! But five years into my doula career, as I turned 40, it all came to a screeching halt.

I did not like the woman I saw in the mirror. She was not the gracefully aging, stylish woman who shopped at fine department stores I had dreamt of becoming. She was gaining weight. Her hair was thinning. Her skin was dull and breaking out. She was exhausted. Her self-talk was ugly.

Who was I becoming, I wondered?

And then I knew ... I was becoming *my mother*—and I didn't like it one bit.

As my mother stared back at me from the mirror, my negative self-talk was in her demeaning voice. And I hated the woman looking back at me, scowling in disapproval.

I had been brainwashed my entire life to believe I wasn't good enough. And I was telling myself the exact same thing. I remember how ugly I felt, standing there in front of the mirror, feeling the knife of self-loathing drive through my soul.

I had struggled with depression and anxiety, especially around my cycle, my entire life. As the symptoms deepened, I became increasingly concerned about my mental health.

People began asking me if I was *"going through the changes."*

I wanted to die.

Literally.

Now, when women talk about this, so many are told, "It's all in your head." And for a few years, I believed it. I mean, I didn't *look* sick. I figured I'd just live with it, as many other women had before me and would after me.

But then came the day when I had had enough—enough of the moodiness, the insomnia, the weight gain, and the skin breakouts. The ups and downs were affecting my work, my relationships, and my family. I knew something had to change.

I made an appointment with my midwife. She prescribed birth control to balance my hormones. I visited my OB. He prescribed hormone replacement to balance my hormones. I didn't fill either script. I called a psychiatrist. She suggested antidepressants to manage my symptoms. No, thank you! I've never been one to rely on prescription medications. (I gave birth to three children without pain meds ... if I could do that, I figured I could do this!)

With no good options in front of me, I found myself wondering what I would do if one of my clients came to me with my symptoms. What would I tell her? And that's when I had an epiphany—I became my own client.

I took a long hard look at my hormone history and my life, beginning with puberty.

I remembered how awful it was, complete with mood swings, unexplained feelings of rage, anxiety, depression, and occasional breakouts. I felt like it would never end.

I thought back to giving birth to my children, and the memories of postpartum depression haunted me. Having been diagnosed with Postpartum Mood Disorder, it was the absolute lowest point of my life. When I had my first son (who was born four weeks early), I was a single mother. My son's father and I only knew each other a short time before we got pregnant. As soon as I told him the news, he broke up with me. I had zero support—no family or friends nearby to help. I came home from the hospital with my tiny little baby to an empty apartment. Money was tight, because I was not entitled to a paid maternity leave. In the days that followed, I also knew I wasn't getting enough sleep or nutrients.

I remembered the anxiety, the loneliness, the fear ... before I knew it, everything started spinning out of control, and my condition spiraled into Postpartum Psychosis. I was delusional. I said strange things and believed even stranger things. I saw and heard things that weren't there.

I tried talking to family and friends about my feelings and thoughts. Nobody understood. My mother told me to "snap out of it!" and, as she would often say, "You wanted a baby; you got a baby." I felt completely alone and uncared for. I had trouble sleeping, I was losing weight at a rapid pace, because I couldn't eat. I wanted to run away. The simplest things, like driving or preparing a meal, became scary and/or hard. It was difficult to take care of myself while taking care of my baby.

I would lie in bed at night planning my own suicide. That's not easy to type, but it's true.

I desperately *wanted* to "snap out of it." Believe me. I *wanted* to enjoy my baby. I wanted to stop the roller coaster in my brain. But I had no idea how. I needed help, and I couldn't find it.

Continuing my reflection, I remembered meeting Colleen at a professional networking event. She had seen a blog article I'd written about postpartum depression, and asked me about my experience. Colleen, who was older than me, then shared her own struggle with postpartum anxiety.

She also warned me that it would all come back in Peri-menopause. I was floored. I left the networking event immediately after she told me, feeling like I had just seen a ghost. I was *scared*.

I drove my car home repeating my mantras. *I will not let that happen to me again. I will beat it this time. Not again.*

I remembered all of these details as I reflected back on my history. And that's when I realized that my hormones have been trying to speak to me throughout ALL of it. I came to the conclusion that I might have Premenstrual Dysphoric Disorder (PMDD) while going through Perimenopause at the same time. The two combined would surely make my symptoms worse—a double whammy. Armed with this new theory, I went back to the Midwife, the Obstetrician, and the Psychiatrist, and presented my case to each of them again. The three were in unanimous agreement that I was right. Their solution? The exact same prescriptions AGAIN! And, again, I declined every one of them.

So, treating myself as I would my own client, I knew a smart place to start would be to take a good, hard look at my lifestyle. Included in that was my mindset and diet.

Being healthy is a lifestyle, and self-care is a BIG part of it. It's about making mindful choices throughout the entire day in order to better care for oneself. I learned that it is through optimal self-care that I am better at everything—my work, as a mother and wife, and as a friend. It's about way more than what I eat and how many yoga classes I can bank in a week. It actually starts the minute I put my feet on the floor every morning, and ends when I rest my head on my pillow, *every single day*.

I also knew I had to focus on nutrition, which can greatly influence Perimenopause and its symptoms. I learned that one of the most important dietary recommendations for all women is to eat organic, whole foods. I ditched the "wine-and-coffee diet," and made an effort to focus on the following diet changes:

Foods to Eliminate from Your Diet	Foods to Include in Your Diet
Refined Sugar	Cruciferous Vegetables
Caffeine and Alcohol	Omega-3 fatty acids
Highly Spicy Foods	Protein
Saturated Fats	Calcium

Next, I knew I needed to get to bed earlier, and when I did, to turn off the TV, shut down the computer, and switch the phone to airplane mode. Studies show that women experiencing hormone fluctuations need seven to eight hours of restful sleep each night if they want to lose weight, improve the appearance of their skin, and get relief from brain fog. So, I worked on getting into bed at the same time every night *and* at the same time as my partner, to improve our relationship at simultaneously. (Plus, as an added bonus, this helps avoid late night snacking and wine!)

Lastly, I would learn to listen to my body through cycle syncing—a valuable tool for better understanding your body, improving sex, and stabilizing your mood. It's a process by which you get to know exactly what's happening in your ovaries, fallopian tubes, and uterus at any given point during the month. This includes watching your cervical fluid for changes, listening to their body's cravings for sex, and paying attention to other symptoms that could flare up during your cycle.

Below, you'll see a chart you can use to track exactly how you're feeling each day, as you really listen to your body.

Reflection Chart: Fill in your answers to the following questions.

What do I do even though I don't want to?

_____

_____

_____

If I were to wave a magic wand, which three things would I change about my life?

_____

_____

_____

Would I feel happy with my progress in one year from today if I were in the same space? Why or why not?

_____

_____

_____

Throughout this entire journey, I have learned so much. I believe if puberty isn't easy, neither will PMS. If PMS is escalated, it can become PMDD. If you have PMDD, you are at a greater risk for Postpartum Mood Disorder. And if you struggle after having a baby, you definitely might struggle through Perimenopause.

I've learned that, despite medical mindset theories around perimenopause being an estrogen-deficiency disease resulting from ovarian failure, it's actually all hormone related. As those hormones change, your body reacts to that change. So, as our hormones fluctuate, so do our moods, because the human brain plays a big part in the hormonal control center and in our body's responses. Essentially, I believe it's not necessarily a hormone "imbalance." It's the body's response to the fluctuation.

I've learned that (and many women are not aware of this) hormones can start to shift as early as 35 years old. Usually, this shifting begins to occur about three to six years before your last period, as the body approaches menopause. During Perimenopause, you still get your period, which could be regular or not.

Perimenopause is very similar to puberty in regard to the similar shifting of hormones. It's also when some women begin to notice the symptoms of hormonal changes, such as menstrual irregularities, breast tenderness, brain fog, insomnia, weight gain, hot flashes or sweats, mood changes, fatigue, and vaginal dryness.

What I most want you to take away from this chapter is that you are NOT alone. You don't have to struggle the way I did. You CAN balance your hormones naturally, using the tips I've shared above. And you CAN feel better.

Nicole Buratti

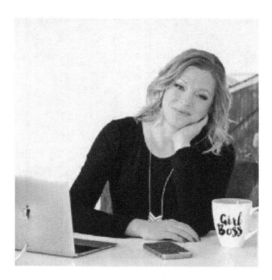

Nicole Buratti is a Certified Women's Health Coach and Registered Yoga Teacher specializing in women's health and bodies. Her passion is in educating, providing understanding, and supporting women who are going through hormonal changes. Her goal is to bring awareness to women about what is happening in their bodies, and to celebrate it with them. You can learn more about her here: sextalkwithnicole.com.

Get Nicole's free gift, her **Hormones Masterclass, designed to get you feeling energized and healthy again,** here: hopebookseries.com/gifts.

Chapter 12

From Broken to Healthy: A Journey of Hope

By Kara Krueger

There is evidence that, before we return to our next lifetime in this amazing realm, we choose. We choose the family that will provide our needed experience. We choose the specific lessons we want to learn, and the growth we want to achieve. We choose the obstacles we want to overcome, and the ways in which we will inspire others.

We make all of these choices in the hopes of making it to the next great chapter of life.

Sometimes, it feels like I had a rather noble day in the Spirit place, when I checked a *bunch* of boxes for this lifetime's lessons!

My childhood felt difficult. From a very young age, I struggled under the weight of being highly intuitive. While it is definitely a gift, it was also challenging to understand and manage, especially without guidance. I spent much of my younger years desperately trying to cope with hard emotions and an acute sense of others' pain. I was not able to determine what belonged to me, and what I was absorbing from those around me. This led to a great deal of anxiety, a lack of confidence, and a feeling of being "different" in a way no one understood.

When it all became too overwhelming, I made the conscious choice to tuck my gifts (and related challenges) into my back pocket, hiding them away. I then began "crashing" into the world far too young—crashing into people, substances, and dangerous situations—all the while seeking out experiences that might somehow curb my innate pain and confusion. I longed for relief ... to feel better while making some sense out of everything going on inside me.

I became a mother in my teens, which helped me get balanced for a bit. But the harshness of my reality soon came full circle, and I surrendered to the idea that I was broken. My children ended up in the care of others close to me during the worst times of my addiction and poor choices (which I was incredibly grateful for).

I didn't plan on living past 30.

It wasn't long before the weight and chaos of my hard choices began taking their toll. I came to understand that I wasn't just dealing with painful events in my childhood and a lack of guidance. I was also combatting unique physical and mental challenges, as well.

An early lack of good nutrition and nutrients fueled my poor health and emotional imbalance. I experienced brief periods of homelessness, and often felt very lost and alone.

It was when my health began declining even further that I finally found a bit of hope.

You see, despite all of the hardships, I had always clung to the deep sense within me that *I am made from something good*. Somehow, I never lost the idea that I *am* connected to the Divine. Even during the worst of times, I was aware of an inner guidance that gently (and sometimes assertively) steered me.

Eventually, it steered me toward the beginning of help and hope.

At age 30, the consequences of my choices led to my probation, which included mandatory treatment. At the treatment center, I looked around me and saw people with stories similar to mine. Hearing about their successes gave me hope, and I was intrigued by the light in their eyes! They helped me realize that I really wasn't unique, which was a vital key to receiving new ideas. This was, then, the beginning of a new chapter of my life, in which I could finally see potential solutions to my brokenness.

But I wasn't done learning the hard lessons, yet. I took one more brief tour in chaos, which ultimately led to time (via the justice system) to sit down, reflect, and work on myself. It was the first time in my life that I allowed myself to believe that I just might make it.

That was in 1995, and I made a commitment to myself to be open to every resource I could find that might benefit my future.

I have never since returned to the lifestyle that had come so close to destroying me.

Over the years, life presented me with so many beautiful offerings, along with endless ways to continue to heal and grow.

I began taking part in Native American teachings and ceremonies, connecting with their spiritual practices. This resonated deeply in me, becoming an integral part of my healing.

I became part of circles of powerful women, which helped me heal many wounds while providing me with so much inspiration. One of these women, a friend and social worker, gifted me counseling, which proved invaluable as we unraveled the places in my childhood that had become so painful and limiting.

My own dedication to healing and change presented me with many opportunities to be present for (and begin helping) others. For the next ten years, I worked in treatment centers helping others who were on similar journeys as mine by developing models of treatment that changed old paradigms. All the while, I took on learning all I could about nutrition. Coming to understand that our body is an incredible creation that continuously work for us, I realized the need to find ways to hear all it asks for. For so long, I hadn't realized the intricate link between foods and supplement therapies and mind/body balance. I learned how to recognize my own body's desire to heal and be in balance. It was in need of some long-overdue attention in order to overcome a lifetime of poor digestion and liver issues. And my mind required its own nutrients to become centered and productive.

So, I decided to go to school for nutrition, and from there, began helping people on even deeper levels with the tools I'd acquired. Not only did I begin teaching classes about nutrition and healthy foods at the treatment centers, but I also started my first nutrition counseling business in 2005.

Thirsty for knowledge and growth, I began working on my mindset, too ... unraveling belief systems that no longer served me. I let go of the belief that my health was someone else's responsibility. I stopped believing I couldn't heal. I learned new ways to "re-landscape" and optimize both my body and my mind. I discovered Epigenetics, which opened floodgates of understanding around life-long health challenges.

All of this has led me to where I am now—in the greatest health of my life!

Looking back to thirty years ago, I realize my life likely looked a waste. It all seemed so hopeless, and the lessons so painful.

But the truth is, going through those exact challenges brought me to all my life *could* be. It brought me to my life's purpose—being a healer! It was these very experiences that led me to becoming a board-certified nutrition counselor and opening Peak Wellness Group, where I now utilize the many tools I learned with my clients to address the multitudinous sides of the healing journey.

If you're struggling now, like I was, please remember that life *is* amazing. Sure, some of the lessons we learn along the way are formidable opponents that demand great strength and courage. Others may only whisper.

All the while, you *can* find reasons to choose more love, be in gratitude, and continue discovering ways to support your own wellness.

When we decide to take just one step in a better direction, we open up opportunities to make incredible progress. We are supported in countless seen and unseen ways. And we carry on!

Wondering how to take that first step?

Let's start easy—consider your answers to the following questions:

What health goals would you like to achieve?

What is the first step you can take toward reaching them?

What will your life look like when you reach these goals—how will it be better?

Who will assist you (friends, support groups, practitioners)?

Once you know the answers to these questions, you can seek guidance to help you through the next chapter of your health and wellness.

You *don't* have to "go it" alone.

Remember:

We often arrive to hard circumstances. If you can shift your mindset to view those circumstances as opportunities for growth, you've already started the work that leads to transformation. The beauty here is that the times that appear least sacred can actually become the most valuable to your purpose!

YOU are in charge of your life. YOU are a powerful Creator.

And you CAN take charge and change direction whenever you wish.

Kara Krueger

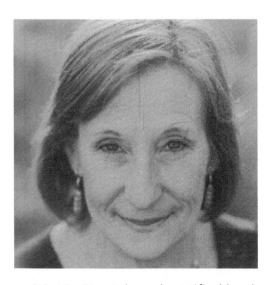

Kara Krueger, BCNC, CNHP, board-certified by the American Naturopathic Medical Certification Board nutrition counselor, certified by the Trinity School of Natural Health, and founder of Peak Wellness Group has been helping her clients take charge of their health since 2005. Passionate about guiding others to achieve balance in body and mind, she utilizes the cutting-edge science of epigenetics and nutrigenomics to assist her clients in living their best lives! Certified by the National Association of Certified Natural Health Professionals, Kara's many years of expertise in the fields of addiction and mental health counseling also support her in furthering her mission of promoting wellness. You can learn more about her here: peakwellnessgroup. com.

What health mysteries are hiding in your genetics? Find out by answering five questions that reveal keys to unlocking potential and optimizing your health. Get Kara's free gift—the **What Health Mysteries Are Hiding in Your Genetics Quiz**—here: hopebookseries.com/gifts.

Chapter 13

The "Natural" Balance—Ending the Struggle with Hormones, for Good!

By Stephanie Lopez Gilmore

I still remember the day I first started my cycle. I was 14 years old when I noticed the blood in the toilet as I was going to the bathroom at school. I was scared and very unprepared. I was too embarrassed to ask my teacher for a pad, or any of the other girls at school (as far as I knew, none of them had gotten theirs yet). Instead, I made a makeshift pad with tissue, and when my mom came to pick me up from school, she took me to the local pharmacy to buy pads.

Now, my story isn't horrible, right? I've heard worse. And I am grateful for that! But what came later was much, much worse. The pain was the worst I have ever experienced. The cramps came with a vengeance, making it feel like someone was ripping open my uterus with a knife and stabbing me in the back. I tried everything: hot packs, Midol, rocking back in forth in the fetal position … but nothing helped.

Because of the debilitating pain, I had to miss school frequently. After a few months, my mother took me to Urgent Care to address the cramps. The doctor recommended I make an appointment with a specialist, so we booked an appointment with a gynecologist. After the awkward probing, I was told that the only thing that can aid in extreme cramp-related pain was birth control pills. My mother hesitated, but then finally agreed to the prescription medication. I remember feeling immediate relief.

Fast-forward 14 years, and I was still taking prescription contraception. Although I didn't know it at the time, for 14 years, I had been putting toxins in my body.

It wasn't until 2018, when I was 28 years old, that I really realized what I had done to my body. It had been eight years since I stopped taking it (my insurance stopped covering it, and because my husband and I had begun talking about starting a family), but I was still dealing with the backlash of them: excess weight gain, painful periods, night sweats, low sex drive, and chest and back acne in my 20's and 30's.

My hormones were out of whack, but I already knew that, thanks to the naturopathic physician who told me in 2010 that my body was a "hostile environment to raise kids" due to my increased level of testosterone. Did I take warning, then? Nope … I wasn't planning on having kids, so I actually thought "Cool, permanent birth control mechanism!"

Well, in 2018, that changed rather abruptly when I experienced painful breast tenderness that lasted almost 10 days. I panicked, thinking I was pregnant. When I saw a gynecologist to get my hormones tested, I was told that the tenderness was a "normal" symptom (I now know she meant of fluctuating hormones), and that things would "regulate out" on their own. I was told there was no need to get tested, and advised to get back on birth control pills.

Let me tell you how frustrating and infuriating it is to go to a specialist seeking answers as to why your body is not functioning properly only to be told that it's "normal" and not to worry. I was brushed off when I asked for hormonal testing and looked at like I was absolutely crazy when I refused the prescription and asked for a natural alternative. I left the office confused, frustrated, and angry that I wasted my afternoon in her office without getting any answers.

Instead of letting the frustration eat me up, I decided to channel it into doing my *own* research on natural alternatives to balance hormones. I wanted to learn as much as I possibly could about hormonal health.

Less than one week later, I was attending a networking event when a colleague of mine handed me a book about balancing hormones, saying she felt I would benefit from it. I had never told her about my hormonal health problems … yet she handed me the key that unlocked the treasure chest holding all the answers I was seeking.

Funny how the universe works, isn't it?

I spent the next nine months researching and trying out various programs and theories on myself. What I discovered was that there are so many symptoms of hormonal imbalances that I hadn't recognized and had blatantly ignored. I learned the symptoms of hormonal imbalance, which include low energy, foggy brain, acne, irregular periods, heavy bleeding, painful periods, moodiness, PMS, depression, headaches, vaginal dryness, weight gain in the mid-section, fibrocystic breasts, breast tenderness (lo and behold!), Endometriosis, fibroids, and thyroid dysfunction.

Over a three-month period, after changing my diet and adding supplements to help regulate my hormones, I noticed a dramatic change in my hormonal health. The first sign of improvement was a reduction in breast tenderness. The second was a dramatic reduction in hormonal acne (which, for a woman in her 30's, was very annoying!). Then I began to notice things that I had honestly stopped thinking about until they were no longer present, like vaginal dryness, night sweats, moodiness, bloating, and finally ... the cramps!

I was so excited—had I created a non-prescription remedy to regulate hormones and reduce symptoms that I thought would never go away?

My life improved dramatically. Even my family noticed a difference in my mood and cycles. My menses improved, going from five days of heavy flow to three medium-to-light days of bleeding.

I couldn't wait to share my excitement with others, and when I did, I began to notice that my friends, colleagues, and clients were all suffering from hormonal imbalances. I desperately wanted to share what I had created to heal myself from my hormonal symptoms with them. So, I took on a handful of clients and tested it out on them. They all experienced improvements, too!

Soon I found myself engaged in conversations with clients and friends around topics and questions like, "What's the color of your menses blood? How often do you have a bowl movement and what's the texture like? What type of body products and laundry detergent do you use?" These conversations became my new norm, and I honestly loved them. I also loved the text messages and calls from women rejoicing about finally losing the 15 stubborn pounds they had gained suddenly … from others rejoicing after having a menstrual cycle for the first time in years without prescription medication … others who were able to reduce PMS symptoms … and it was all I needed to hear to know that I have truly found my purpose.

Looking back, I am so grateful for that doctor's visit back in 2018, when I left so frustrated. Because that is the day I decided to take my health back into my own hands—and it resulted in finding my life's passion.

Since that day, I have helped many women cycle off prescription contraceptives and medications like metformin, and avoid procedures like DNC and hysterectomy. Knowing that I am helping them regain confidence, energy, and vitality is so rewarding!

To help you begin doing the same, here are six steps to optimizing your hormones:

Step 1: Take time to tap into your body.

Too often, we are so disconnected from our bodies. We ignore our symptoms. We power though to get tasks done, only to take note when something becomes debilitating. Take the time *now*. Here's one of my favorite methods:

Find a quiet place to sit without distractions. Sit or lay down and close your eyes. Focus on your breath for five inhales and exhales to calm the body and tune out other thoughts. Next, complete a mental full-body scan, starting from your head and going to your toes. Notice if anything seems tense, if there is any pain anywhere, or heat radiating. Tap into how your body feels at the moment. Are you alert or tired? Do you feel happy or upset?

Step 2: Reflect on how you feel during your menstrual cycle.

Do you notice that your energy levels are low more often than not? Do you feel bloated? Do you tend to get moody around your cycle? Are you experiencing pain? What other symptoms arise?

Step 3: Talk with your doctor.

Now that you understand the symptoms, the next step is to start a conversation with your doctor regarding the symptoms. If your doctor is not very receptive (which is unfortunately the case for many of my clients), then find a naturopathic doctor who specializes in women's hormonal health (or reach out to me).

Step 4: Get tested.

There are a lot of hormone tests out there, so finding the right one for you is key (my personal recommendation is the DUTCH test, which I recommend to all my clients).

Step 5: "Let food be thy medicine."

One of the best ways to balance your hormones naturally is with food. I know … it's not an easy task for many, as we tend to have a strong connection with food. But it *is* necessary to get back to a balanced state.

One of the most effective ways to start the healing process with food is by following the Elimination Diet, in which you eliminate the following foods that tend to affect your hormones the most: red meat, caffeine, alcohol, sugar, dairy, grains, and fruit.

Step 6: Get support.

A coach can guide you through the process of healing your hormones, which can be difficult at times. Having an expert by your side, guiding you, answering your questions, and supporting you through this change is worth the investment!

The bottom line is that you do NOT have to suffer through symptoms caused by hormonal imbalance. Night sweats, hot flashes, low libido, cramps, PMS, PCOS and Endometriosis can be eliminated/healed with diet and lifestyle changes—in other words, with a natural approach instead of with harmful prescription medications and procedures like a DNC or hysterectomy. Optimal health and hormonal happiness is within your reach!

Stephanie Lopez Gilmore

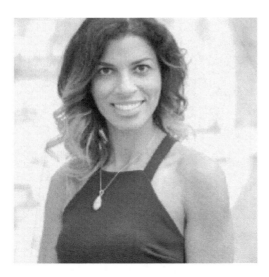

Stephanie Lopez Gilmore is a Hormonologist health coach who studies women's hormonal health. She battled with her own hormonal health problems as a teen and as an adult before making it her mission to offer her clients a holistic solution to their hormonal problems. To learn more, go to stephanielopezgilmore.com.

Get Stephanie's free gift, her Hormonal Health Tool Kit: Quiz, Cheat Sheet, and Self-Care Guide, designed to aid you get you on the path to healing, naturally, here: hopebookseries.com/gifts.

Chapter 14
Believe

By Christi Davis

Nothing happens by accident as we create our destiny.

When I was 26 years old, I jokingly wished out loud that I could be struck with a condition to control my eating and weight. I was getting married that year, and despite my efforts, could not lose weight. I struggled with portion control, along with my ultimate downfall since childhood: sweets. Two years later, in the fall of 2001, my wish came true.

After several MRI's of my brain, various neurological tests, and finally, a spinal tap that sealed the diagnosis, the neurologist said, "You have multiple sclerosis."

This was right after 9/11—which shook me to the core. I was living just two hours away from the city at the time, but had grown up within an hour from there. My husband and I also stayed in NYC for our honeymoon in 1999 and dined at Windows on the World on the 106th floor of the World Trade Center—also known as North Tower, Building One. The thought of what occurred that day is horrifying and had a huge impact on me. Although I did not know anyone directly affected by 9/11, it truly sickened me to comprehend what happened there. I was terrified about our future.

Needless to say, receiving the MS diagnosis during this time was a difficult blow, and "scared out of my mind" is an understatement. I was only 28, and newly married. I was just getting my career going (ironically, working for a motorized wheelchair manufacturer). I immediately thought the worst, and was plagued by questions: would I succumb to this disease I knew nothing about? Would I end up in one of the very wheelchairs that were going through the production line at my work? Would my husband still want to be married to me if I became disabled?

Should we take the notion of having a family off the table? Should we sell our newly built house and find a one level ranch?

Outside the neurologist's office, I immediately called my mom in an utter panic. I was able to take a few days off work and head to my parents for a long weekend. Being with family really helped ground and focus me on what I *could* control. I knew if I let myself go any further down that "what if?" path, it would not end well. My family helped me embrace the power of positivity, and I have held onto that belief system ever since.

Multiple Sclerosis is a chronic autoimmune disease that affects the central nervous system. The myelin sheath that covers and protects the brain breaks down, causing lesions or plaques. As a result, the electrical impulses from the brain do not flow smoothly, resulting in issues with vision, balance, mobility, muscle control, and other basic body functions. Each individual with MS has his or her own unique symptoms and journey with the disease. I have the Remitting Relapsing version and stay mostly in remission (which I am hugely grateful for, as it is the least severe of the three forms of MS).

The initial symptom I experienced was vertigo—a constant feeling of dizziness. Shortly after, optic neuritis, a key indicator of MS, set in my right eye. This inflammation of the optic nerve causes visual field loss, loss of color vision, and eye pain. It also limits peripheral vision. The best way I can describe this condition is to imagine having holes in your vision and dramatic color reduction. (So strange, when my other eye was completely normal.) It can last a few weeks to several months. I also felt perpetually stuck in a sort of fog, and was constantly fatigued. And to top it off, I was also dealing with numbness and constant tingling in my feet and legs.

A friend of mine recommend I see a Holistic Healing Practitioner who practiced Iridology (diagnosis by examination of the iris of the eye). I did, and was more than a little surprised when she basically recalled my entire health history without my divulging a single bit of information. (She also called me out on eating entirely too much ice cream. I remember thinking, "Whoa ... how does she know that?!)

When she recommended a "diet sans"—no gluten, dairy, pork, beef, or sugar—I thought she was insane! But, since I had heard how she helped others, actually healing many disease states, I figured it was worth a try.

I struggled with what to make (back then, the gluten-free options were less than desirable ... pasta, which had always been one of my favorites having grown up in an Italian family, was like mush!), and I definitely got stuck on all the things I could NOT eat. As hard as it was, I stuck with it (not to say I was strict about it, consistently, but I did always gravitate back to it when I stopped feeling on point). And to my surprise, I felt *clearer*—like the fog lifted. I knew my practitioner was definitely on to something!

During all of this, my husband and I still wanted to have a family. We diligently researched our options in connection with my diagnosis. I even joined an online support group, and received some very negative feedback around our decision to have children. I was called "selfish," "ignorant," and "immoral." The "haters" said there was too much risk in passing on my disease to my children, which would then burden them. But in all our research, and in consulting my neurologist, we learned that the risk of my children inheriting it was extremely low. And from where I was standing, I wasn't willing to allow the disease to destroy our dream of having a family.

Doctors did recommend that I go off my medications during pregnancy, as there were associated risks. So I did, and family planning began. We had our son in November of 2003 and our daughter in April 2005. Once I was done breastfeeding, I started taking my medication, and have continued to consistently to this day.

Having our children further grounded me in the reality of how important it is to focus on my health. I knew if I was not well, they would pay the price. As the saying goes, "You cannot pour from an empty pitcher." So, my children effectively drove my inner mission to maximize my health and thrive at all levels. After my daughter was born, I got a full handle on portion control for the first time in my life. (Honestly, it stemmed from a "forced nature," really ... since my kiddos were only 17 months apart, I had no time to complete a meal!) But it also made me realize that I didn't need to finish my overfilled plate of food, because I would actually get full about one half to three quarters way through my meal. Eye-opening to say the least!

I'm proud to say I have maintained my current weight (which is 20 pounds less than the day I was married) since 2005!

In 2011, a year after my dad's passing, I faced my second bout of optic neuritis. I was admitted to the hospital for IV steroids to help improve my vision. I also knew it was time to make more changes to my diet and lifestyle. While I had always worked out and followed my diet protocol, it was a bit off and on, and at this point, I knew it was time to be more consistent.

Then, my mom was diagnosed with cancer in 2014. I flew to Florida (where she was vacationing) because she ended up having to undergo an emergency craniotomy. Scary stuff, to say the least. I believe this stress triggered my MS symptoms, the main one being the "MS Hug," where your entire abdominal circumference goes numb. More scary stuff. In light of mom's stage four lung cancer diagnosis (which spread to her brain), I very quickly learned about organic eating and how food can truly heal. So, I began cooking organic, vegetable-based meals for us. I went for runs and did strength training workouts while she rested. My MS Hug improved every day, and was just about gone when we came back home seven days later.

Thanks to more research on my brother's part, Mom was put on a diet consisting of organic juicing, organic foods, dairy/gluten/sugar-free foods, specific supplements, and daily nutritional protocols. Her tumors began to shrink, and that is when I truly made the complete shift in how we ate as a family. While yes, eating organically *is* expensive, I consider it an investment in our health—the most valuable thing in the world to me!

During my mom's second round of chemo and brain radiation, her cancer took a turn for the worse, and she passed away. There are so many things we wish we could have done for her, and it has made a forever mark on me. Still, I know if she were still with us, she would be so proud of our commitment to holistic eating. While I do still endure some minor flare-ups from time to time, I'm happy to report that I have remained almost exclusively in remission since my diagnosis back in 2001!

Late in 2018, I experienced an inner calling to pursue my passion around food, nutrition, fitness, and health. Keep in mind almost 20 years prior, I had obtained a degree in Nutrition while never turning it into a career. I knew it was "now or never," so I started by taking a class called "The Power of Food" through our county night school. The woman teaching the course was a Certified Health Coach, and she was wonderful. The content was awesome, and I realized how much I already knew because of all of my previous research surrounding my disease and mom's cancer. This excited me, and I ended up attending the Health Coach Institute, which applies the integrative nutrition approach that I wholeheartedly believe in along with the game-changing concept of Lifestyle Habit Change.

As a Certified Health and Life Coach, I now offer those individuals struggling with autoimmune health and weight loss issues the tools to start thriving and enjoying their life to the fullest potential! I work with clients to help them implement permanent habit changes that will set them up for long-term success.

I have chosen to share my story and journey because it ultimately guided me through the process of untapping my life's passion and destiny to help others struggling with the same types of health challenges that I have. I am more motivated than ever to make a difference in so many lives. The most important piece of changing our health is to BELIEVE that it's possible!

Christi Davis

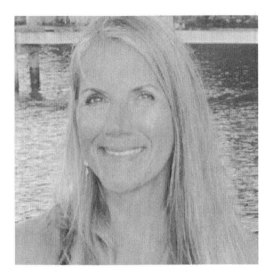

Christi Davis, founder of Christi Health Coach, is a self-proclaimed "nutrition nerd." Certified Health Coach through the Health Coach Institute (accredited through the International Coaching Federation), she specializes in autoimmune wellness, helping people reclaim their energy and confidence in the face of health challenges while guiding them in living their absolute best life. Join her private Facebook group—Autoimmune Wellness and Whole Body Nutrition—for tips, recipes, and challenges. Learn more about her here: christihealthcoach.com.

And, get Christi's free gift, her Autoimmune Friendly Cookbook, consisting of 15 flavor-packed, autoimmune-friendly recipes that will please your family and friends, too! hopebookseries.com/gifts.

Chapter 15
Choosing the Path That Offers a Bridge

By Deni Carruth

Imagine morning sickness so bad you can't even keep your own saliva down. That was me! Six weeks pregnant with my second child, I lay curled up on the floor by the toilet. The last call I placed to my OBGYN resulted in orders to go immediately to the ER for admission.

They couldn't get me to my room fast enough. Once there, I waited for an IV for dehydration, and then an injection to stop the nausea and vomiting.

That's when my life changed.

The nurse rolled me slightly forward from my side. When I felt the needle enter my right buttock, my leg began to shake uncontrollably. The pain was unbearable! Even now, remembering that moment brings a lump to my throat.

My leg relaxed when she removed the needle, but the pain did not stop. I was assured it would, but it didn't. In fact, that was the beginning of what seemed to be a never-ending journey of pain I'll never forget.

When the pain, numbness, and fear didn't subside as my baby continued growing inside me, my OB referred me to a neurologist. Then another. They provided little hope, and basically told me that my profession as a fitness specialist was in jeopardy due to the physical component of my profession. Having previously overcome a bout with chronic pain, I had committed myself to bringing safe and purposeful movement to others. Unwilling to settle, my OB referred me to a third neurologist.

I remember sitting in his office so clearly. He believed my sciatic nerve had been damaged. He shared that he had only ever seen two cases (he called them "direct hits") in which that particular medication was (possibly) injected into the muscle or nerve. In the first, the woman's muscle tissue was "eaten away," leaving a baseball-sized hole in her buttock. She maintained some function. In the second, the woman had no visible marks, but functionally, she had almost no use of her leg. Not promising.

Medication was out of the question because of my baby. But this doctor's mindset was much different than the others: he was *with* me. He had a "What can WE do?" point of view, instead of telling me what I couldn't do, which gave me hope.

The answer? A TENS unit! Non-traditional, yes, but possibly very effective.

I have to tell you, that unit practically became a part of my body! I wore it *all* the time. It lessened the intensity and duration of my pain as well as the frequency of pain awareness. And I was SO happy, because it gave me the means to stay in my profession! I continued to teach my signature exercise classes (with my hubby's help in demonstrations) and see one-on-one clients.

After my daughter was born, my doctor added in some traditional medicine. I was good with that—caring for my baby and helping others with movement and function was my goal.

I was learning how to be the chooser of my life, and how important that really was. Because at any given moment, we get to *choose* what's best for us. We can decide to live life as fully as it can be in each moment.

No guilt. No shame.

I was grateful, and still on purpose. But I was not done being challenged.

Looking back at pictures of my baby shower, I realized that something else was going on with my body. In order to sit for any length of time, I intentionally sat on one "cheek" and crossed my legs, which rotated my pelvis while twisting my torso in the opposite direction. This way, it would appear like I was sitting straight. I know. Sounds crazy, but it's what I did to cope and appear "normal."

This "subtle" twisting of my spine created a *pronounced* curvature called "postural scoliosis"—which, thank goodness, is reversible.

I realized I had caused *additional* pain for myself, sitting in a way that created muscle imbalances and tension in my back.

In the '80s, when all this was occurring, chiropractic care was still very non-traditional. I had both good and not-so-good experiences with chiropractors before, but I was ready to take the risk again, as I really needed to get some relief in my back. I had done for myself all that I knew to do based on my training and experience with traditional and corrective exercise, and I knew it was time to *choose* to seek more help.

After several regular visits with my third (yes, the third was the charm, again) chiropractor, we had an honest conversation. He told me, while he *could* treat my symptoms of this (new) misalignment in my spine, he could *not* treat the problem that was causing me to sit twisted for relief, which was nerve damage.

He encouraged me to not give up. He felt it critical that I seek pain management help, and after much discussion, he informed me that a world-renown neurosurgeon (who, by the way, was the inventor of the TENS unit) had a pain management facility RIGHT IN OUR TOWN! What?!

There was hope again!

I remember my first appointment and evaluation at the Shealy Institute for Pain and Depression Rehabilitation so vividly.

I stood at the front desk, noticing several large crystals placed around the room. A picture of "healing energy" handprints hung on the wall. I immediately wondered if they were treatment techniques used in the facility.

I was a little bit concerned, because I wasn't sure if those techniques were in line with my Christian belief system. So I inquired, and the response I received highlighted an incredible amount of research that had been performed there in the name of one goal: to help people heal without surgery or loads of medication being the first or only choices.

I was fascinated, and yet, I admit ... a little uncomfortable, still.

But the appointment ended up giving me such hope! Suddenly, there were new possibilities open to me. The people of Shealy genuinely cared for ME.

Dr. Roger Cady, who became my attending doctor, asked me two questions that day that I'll never forget:

1) Was I a visual person?

2) When I visualize myself, what am I doing?

I closed my eyes and replied, "I'm running." To which he replied, "And so you will."

BOOM!

I wasn't even a runner. I didn't even jog! But suddenly, I knew that there was hope for me to do whatever I could imagine, *if I chose to.*

Before I left, Dr. C. Norman Shealy himself came in to see me. He encouraged me and informed me of their style of non-surgical rehabilitation. He sealed the hope within me that they would do whatever they could to help me, as long as I was willing to help myself.

Hold the phone. Read that last sentence again.

This program wasn't about them doing things "to" me, while I sat around waiting for my body to heal.

This was about working together to rehabilitate me as a whole person.

Almost in tears, I got home from that appointment and literally fell to my knees, so very grateful for the opportunity God had laid before me.

Once again, I was in a position of *choice.* I prayed about it, and felt very comfortable moving forward.

I chose their out-patient program.

After some time (and no, there were no crystal therapies), it was decided that I needed their intensive program.

Both Dr. Shealy and Dr. Cady made it possible for me to make the best decision for me. It was *my* choice. They were going to help me, and I would move forward.

To this day, I cannot thank them enough.

If you can relate to my story, you may be in that "darker" place, right now.

I want you to know there IS hope, and I can walk you through an exercise right now to help you begin your healing journey. Ready?

Step 1: Take a deep breath.

Maybe you have a desire for prevention of, or a solution to, a painful health path.

Your mindset will determine your journey. It's critical that you're able to see what's on the other side of your current situation. So, close your eyes. What will you be doing when you reach the other side of your health concern? Visualize yourself doing whatever it is you long to do.

Step 2: Take a deep breath.

Are excuses stopping you? Are reasons calling you?

It's important to understand your "why" behind your desired transition. I had to be "whole" again because of who I was, what I was called to do, and the mother I knew I wanted to BE.

Step 3: Take a deep breath.

Who do you need to be in this situation? What part of you can you draw on to make best choices for yourself?

With "connectedness" being number five of my top five strengths, everything happens for a … purpose! I had to tap into that. And with "belief" being my third, I knew once I dug in, I wouldn't—couldn't—waver. I was IN!

Step 4: Take a deep breath.

What's possible?

You may think, *anything is!* You may think, *nothing is.* And now we're back to mindset.

Remember, there is hope! If you get nothing more from this, please take that with you! Hope might just be right around the corner from you, like it was for me, and you don't even know it. Being fully present and willing to make choices for yourself can open doors, reveal paths, and offer bridges for purposeful steps forward.

Step 5: Take a deep breath.

There can be JOY in the pain of the process.

I forgave the nurse for what happened to me. I knew there was more than my body that was healing. My mind. My spirit. Even my purpose.

Even though some of the hands-on techniques in therapy were painful, they allowed a release. An openness for blood, oxygen, and healing to take place. And healing DID take place.

My experience at the Shealy Institute was nothing short of incredible!

Much to my surprise, even more blessings were coming my way.

One day, I received a call from Dr. Cady asking if I'd have an "opportunity conversation" with him and the head physical therapist. It was an invitation to come on board as an exercise therapist! Whatever I didn't know, they would teach me. Whatever I knew, I would share with them. We would work together in a new way.

And we did, for over three years!

This beautiful opportunity came from such a painful place, and I couldn't help but be grateful.

And here I stand … on the other side.

I always say, "Choose a path that offers a bridge." A bridge can represent so many things, and a safe way of passage to the other side is just one of them. I saw my path as a way for me to feel and be whole again. I saw the Shealy Institute as the bridge that would get me there.

I embarked on a safe passage that would keep me focused and proactive in my own healing process.

And YOU can do the same.

Deni Carruth

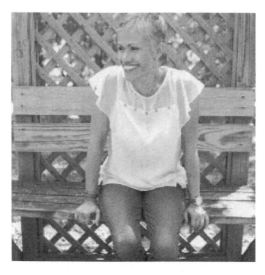

Deni Carruth is a fitness expert and nutrition and life coach who helps women create a lifestyle they can live with ease and JOY. She's a lifestyle strategist who works with the whole of who you are, for results across your life. When Deni isn't working, she's creating ... connections, friendships, graphics, journals, and music. She loves movement, bridges, benches, fresh air, and random rain showers. Oh, and popcorn! Anything forensics has become a "must watch" on TV, and you might find her in a movie that makes her laugh, cry, or grip her seat. You can learn more about her here: denicarruth.com.

Deni's gift to you: "**Choose Change**," a readiness questionnaire with results insights. Get it HERE: hopebookseries.com/gifts.

Chapter 16

Finding Courage in the Darkness of Fear

By Merilee Ford

There I was, sitting in *another* doctor's office, waiting for another test result ... hoping beyond hope for some kind of answer. The doctor came in and said my blood work "looked good." He explained how postpartum mood changes are "normal," and said I was "just fine."

But I wasn't.

At this point in my life, I was no stranger to overcoming obstacles. However, as an adult and new mom, I had set expectations for my life, and things were not going as planned. In fact, they would actually get worse than I ever could have imagined.

As a child, I faced some tough hurdles. But I was successful in my schooling, and ultimately found a job I loved. I got married, and was excited to start my family.

During this time of my life, I spent most of my time outside rock climbing, canyoneering, and enjoying other types of outdoor adventure.

But everything began to change about five weeks after I had my first baby; he became very sick with parainfluenza, and I became acutely aware of anything that could make him sicker. I took constant note of any changes in his health, and of what I perceived as outside dangers. I struggled like this for about nine months, until finally, things felt like they were getting better.

But when I was 34 weeks pregnant with my second child, I was diagnosed with Melanoma—one of the few cancers that can spread to a baby in utero. Surgeries would be required to remove the rest of the Melanoma and my lymph nodes, and to determine whether or not the cancer had spread to other parts of my body or to my baby.

The Oncologist informed me that they could only wait four more weeks to deliver. That month of waiting was incredibly challenging as I became obsessively aware of things that could cause cancer.

My anxiety turned into panic disorder and obsessive-compulsive disorder during and after my third pregnancy. Even though I *knew* these difficult postpartum disorders existed, I had no idea how hard living with them could be. It got so bad, in fact, that I couldn't leave my house for months at a time. I was intensely afraid of chemicals, germs, diseases … of anything and everything that could cause harm. I had panic attacks several times a day, triggered even by loud noises or scents. There were times when it was hard for me to handle objects in my own house. It was difficult for me to cook meals or change diapers, and sometimes, it was even hard for me to hold my kids. When they brought home projects from school that they had made with their sweet little hands, I couldn't bring myself to touch them.

I was trying so hard to keep my family safe that my actions became irrational. The hardest part was that I knew they were irrational, but that awareness didn't change my physiological responses. I couldn't even handle grocery shopping, eating at a restaurant, or taking my kids to the swimming pool. I couldn't enjoy my favorite hobbies, like soccer, anymore, and I wondered if I ever would again.

These relentless, obsessive thoughts and extreme panic were life altering. Even though soccer has always been a huge part of my life, during this time, I had to force myself out of the house to get to games. And when I was able to do that, my mind was consumed the entire time by the potential toxins, germs, and bloodborne diseases I could be bringing back home. I would put my shoes in a plastic bag in the garage. I would take very long showers to make sure I was clean enough to be around my family, and I would wash my clothes immediately.

I was, to put it bluntly, terrified.

On top of these issues, I also found myself battling chronic mononucleosis (mono) and fatigue. There were times when it was literally hard for me to lift my arms to wash my hair, climb the stairs, and open the deadbolt on the front door. I was diagnosed with Crohn's Disease, Rheumatoid Arthritis, Hypothyroidism, Hormone Imbalance, and Chronic Fatigue Syndrome. Doctors offered no solutions or real help.

It was years later that I learned what I was really dealing with: Epstein Barr Virus. Like so many others, I had been mis-diagnosed with countless other conditions.

My life had been reduced to basic survival mode, and I felt completely lost.

All of this took a toll on my husband and kids, as well. It was difficult for others to understand what I was going through. I visited so many doctors and spent thousands of dollars just to be prescribed more medication. In fact, I tried everything suggested to me: medication, therapy, hormone therapy, psychiatry, and genetic testing. Some of these things were helpful in their own way, but did nothing to solve the root problem of my condition. This went on for several years, while time and time again, I ended up right back where I had started. I knew instinctively that I didn't have all the answers, and I continued to get worse.

I would have given *anything* to make it all go away. I would have done anything to feel happy and peaceful ... to be the healthy mom my kids deserved. And I felt guilty, too, because I thought I should have been able to solve the problem. I believed there was something even more wrong with me, because I couldn't just "snap out of it." Many people told me I just needed more faith. Or, if I just *decided* to be happy, I would be ... that I could make it all go away. No one was harder on me than I was on myself, but it was still absolutely devastating to hear these things from the people in my life. Even though I consciously understood that people simply couldn't comprehend what it feels like to live in such intense fear every moment of your life, it didn't make it any easier.

All of this took a terrible toll on my mind and body.

Then, one night, I came to the harsh realization that there was nothing else I could do. I resigned myself to living the rest of my life the way I was. It was a horrible moment.

I felt like I was trapped in a dark box—sometimes, I could see a tiny light, but others, I couldn't. I knew there was a way out, and it *seemed* like it should be simple! But no matter how hard I tried, I could not break free.

As I wrestled with those thoughts, I wondered if my family would be better off without me. I felt like a burden ... worthless and ashamed.

I saw an ad for a suicide hotline.

I dialed the number, and hung up immediately. I dialed again. And hung up again.

I was afraid they might take my kids from me, or punish me in some way for calling. But I didn't know what else to do. I fought those fears and called anyway—and I am *so* glad I did.

I connected with a Maternal Mental Health Therapist who really understood what I was going through. She provided me with immediate help and support. She also put me in touch with a nurse practitioner who helped me explore the effect of nutrition on my health challenges.

The next few years comprised the turning point of my life. It wasn't easy, and it wasn't quick, but it changed everything.

I spent a long time in therapy learning different coping skills, but for some reason, was never able to fully apply them. Meanwhile, I began to treat the Epstein Barr Virus. I didn't realize that build-up from toxins, heavy metals, and stress were causing damage to my organs and adrenal glands. In fact, my body was so overwhelmed, it became unable to absorb nutrients, detoxify, manage hormone levels, or build an immune system effectively. Even the healthy food choices, changes in diet, exercise, and mental coping techniques I tried were overwhelming my body. All of this affected me mentally, as well; it was hard to concentrate, think clearly, and find my way out of the fog. It became clear how much this also contributed to my anxiety.

Once I began "connecting the dots" between my physical, mental, and emotional health, I started to heal.

I learned that I needed to move out the old before bringing in the new. I learned how to heal my detox pathways with the right nutrition, and my Epstein Barr with the right supplements. I developed an awareness for things that could be contributing to the illness, and through my own education, I discovered how to ask for the appropriate tests and care from my doctors. I also began to implement coping strategies for my stress and anxiety in a way that worked for me and my busy family life.

It was amazing to see how things began changing for me once my organs and body began healing and functioning properly again. Layers began to peel away, and everything—the fatigue, sensitivities to scents and noises, fear, pain, hopelessness—all seemed to get a little bit quieter. And then, I was finally able to implement some of the coping techniques I'd learned and explore other methods of healing.

I hadn't expected healing my body physically to have such a profound effect on my mental health! And I had no idea that I could live a life with so much peace and joy.

I learned that health is different for everyone. There is no "one-size-fits-all" approach to wellness, because there are countless different factors that come into play.

When the nurse practitioner who helped me on my journey encouraged me to share everything I'd learned with others who, like me, really needed help, I began researching health and wellness coaching. And I knew without a doubt that it was the culmination of everything in my life, and what I was meant to do.

I never wanted anyone to feel as lost and hopeless as I did. And I knew my own struggles and healing journey could serve others. I knew I could truly make a difference.

Now, as a Wellness Coach myself, it is my mission to be an advocate for my clients, helping them to connect each part of their wellness, and make lasting habit changes.

To anyone who feels hopeless, lost, or desperate for answers, I want you to know you are *not* alone. I was there, too.

But healing *is* possible, and that there *are* answers out there.

The transformation I experienced would not have been possible if I hadn't taken the first step: reaching out for the right help. Yes, it is one of the hardest and scariest parts of the journey, but you never know what is on the other side.

If you are where I was—struggling to understand what is happening with your health—please know that you are not broken, and it's *not* your fault. You are coping the best way you know how.

Now, it is time to shift those coping strategies to those that will serve you better in your healing.

The first step? Get help. You do NOT have to go it alone any longer.

Merilee Ford

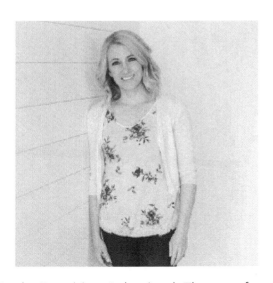

Merilee Ford, Cognitive Behavioral Therapy for OCD and Anxiety and Certified Life and Health Coach is trained in The Advanced Transformational Coaching Method. With a master's degree in Interpersonal Relationships and a bachelor's degree in Psychology, her trainings and programs are based on cutting-edge psychology, brain science, and integrative nutrition. You can learn more about her here: connectthedotshealthcoach.com.

Get Merilee's free gift, a free breakthrough session to help you find clarity to move forward, here: hopebookseries.com/gifts. Merilee will talk with you about your individual needs and struggles, and you'll leave the call with a personalized roadmap to healing just for you!

Chapter 17

Reversing Infertility, Conceiving Naturally, and FINALLY Becoming a Mommy!

By Kela Robinson Smith

I will never forget the night I sat out on my patio and cried. I was 36 years old, and *so* ready to be a mom … but my period had started again, and my hopes of having the family I had always wanted slipped a little further away.

Everyone had said it would be "easy." "Oh, you're in good shape," they said. "You eat healthy. You'll have no problems getting pregnant."

Yet month after month for years, it was always the same: wishing, waiting, trying, and … nothing. We had visited doctors, taken fertility drugs, and undergone invasive procedures. Nothing was working, and I felt like my heart was breaking.

 Why couldn't I get pregnant? What if it was too late? Why me, God?

I was doing all the right things (or so I thought). I was active and "healthy." I exercised militantly. I ate Lean Cuisine for dinner and watched my weight. I was timing my ovulation. Nothing was physically wrong with me, yet no one could tell me *why* I wasn't conceiving. I think that was the most frustrating part. At least when you're sick, a doctor can evaluate, diagnose, and treat you. But I had no answers.

Things got worse before they got better. I was so mad that I wasn't getting pregnant, I began to self-sabotage. I started working out even more and eating worse. It only took a few months of feeling more miserable than ever before I knew I couldn't live that way any longer. I knew things had to change, one way or another, or I would never have the family I so desperately wanted.

Coupled with the fact that I was sick and tired of everyone telling me I was "fine" and recommending all kinds of things that didn't work, I finally came to realize that I had a choice: I could stay stuck in "victim mode," relying on doctors who weren't helping and procedures that weren't working, or I could take my fertility into my own hands. I could change my habits and implement new practices that would make me healthy from the inside out, increasing my chances of conception. I chose the latter, knowing no matter what happened, I would be better off than I was when I started. I could lead a more productive, happier life.

And it was during that exact time that I also had an epiphany. I had worked in the health and wellness industry for years. I had extensive experience helping my clients with all sorts of challenges, from weight loss to detox to strengthening their bodies. And I had been a personal trainer for many years.

In other words, *I already had the knowledge inside me*. I just had to pull it out.

And that's when I started really examining what I was eating.

I began researching, cooking, and experimenting. I began studying how to use food as medicine to heal my body from within, which I hoped would reverse my infertility naturally. I became super intentional about only consuming foods that would work with my body instead of against it—those that would put my body into optimal state for conception (without sacrificing taste or a ton of time!).

Determined to learn EVERYTHING I could about how to use food as medicine to get pregnant, I even went back to school, obtaining four certifications in health and wellness coaching. And I implemented everything thing I learned—all of the new habits, techniques, and practices—into my life as a new *way* of life.

And that's when everything changed.

I was able to put my body into optimal state for conception, and I FINALLY got pregnant—not once, but twice—naturally!

And as if that wasn't amazing enough, the added bonus is now that I know what foods work with my body and not against it, I am in the best shape of my life in my 40's.

This is the journey that also led me to becoming a certified fertility and hormones coach,

because I am so absolutely passionate about my findings. I want to help as many women as I can avoid the heartwrenching struggle I went through to have a baby. There *is* an easier way. There *is* hope. And I've made it my mission to shout that hope out to the world!

To that end, I'm so excited to share five of the tops keys I discovered for putting your body into the optimal state for pregnancy. Here we go!

Tip 1 - Avoid processed foods. Sounds simple enough, right? The thing is, you might not realize exactly how bad packaged food really is, so you might not avoid it as much as you need to. Your body actually recognizes processed foods as toxins. Most are made with GMO's (genetically modified organisms) and are so full of sugar and toxins that they cause your body to fight against itself. Plus, the more you eat them, the more addicted you become, creating a vicious cycle that leaves you searching for your next "high." This is why it is so important to avoid them altogether.

Tip 2 - Focus on whole food nutrition. Once you've eliminated processed foods from your diet, it's time for whole food nutrition. What does that mean, exactly? Eat only the foods that don't come from a package, like:

- Fresh organic vegetables.

- Lean meat.

- Healthy fats.

- Nuts and seeds.

- Fruits.

- Fresh or dried herbs and spices.

When you do, you'll train your body not to crave the sugar in processed foods. And as an added bonus, you'll be naturally satisfied, so you don't feel so hungry all the time.

Tip 3 - Drink .67x your body weight in water every day. I know—it seems like a *lot*, doesn't it? But the reality is that our body is 60% water, and every system in our body uses water to function. Once you become dehydrated, your body shuts down, and all systems stop … especially the baby-making ones! Drinking the right amount of water will lubricate your joints, organs, muscles, and cells, and will leave your skin plump, hair shiny, gut balanced, digestion running smoothly, and immune system functioning properly. Even better, it'll keep your baby-making hormones happy!

Tip 4 - Manage and eliminate your stress. When you are stressed (whether intentionally or not), your body produces cortisol and goes into "fight or flight" response mode. And when that happens, your baby-making abilities shut down, because your body considers it unsafe to create and carry life. (This is one that really affected my ability to get pregnant, too.) Here are some ways to reduce stress:

- Meditate daily.

- Utilize deep breathing exercises.

- Commit to unwavering self-care and devotion.

Tip 5 - Sleep well. This is another one that hindered me while I thought I was doing everything right! Make sure you get six to eight hours of good quality sleep per night. During this time of rest, your body repairs, recovers, rebuilds, detoxes, and resets, all of which are necessary for creating life. Some ways to make sure you are getting amazing, deep sleep are by:

- Implementing a "power down" hour before bed to unplug, unwind, and reconnect to your spouse or partner.

- Making your bedroom cool and dark.

- Keeping a gratitude journal beside your bed for reflection and appreciation for all your blessings.

All five of these tips helped me put my body into an optimal state for conception, and I teach women all over the world how to use them to do the same. Not only am I living proof that they work, but I truly believe they have helped thousands of women to have babies, and that is what I want for you!

I want you to know that you CAN get pregnant naturally, even if you've been told you may not ever be able to. Start to-day, by following the tips above. You are now empowered to take powerful action to make your dreams of having a child a reality!

Kela Robinson Smith

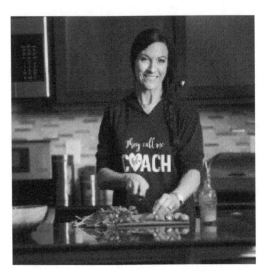

Kela Smith has an extensive background as a professional fitness trainer, wellness educator, and author. To date, she has published two books: The Complete Hormone Puzzle Cookbook and The Hormone Puzzle Method for solving infertility, as well as an online course by the same name. Kela also holds four distinct qualifications as a Certified Holistic Health & Wellness Coach. She realized her dream of creating a virtual holistic health and wellness practice and helps women all over the world solve these issues. As the creator of the Hormone Puzzle Method, Kela helps her clients learn how to cycle sync so they have pleasant periods, boosted fertility, happy hormones, hotter sex lives, and greater creativity, productivity, and wellbeing at work. You can learn more about her here: kelahealthcoach.com.

Download Coach Kela's free gift—a mini fertility plan—here: hopebookseries.com/gifts.

It consists of four breakfasts, four lunches, and four dinners, all of which are nutritious, delicious, and proven to help reverse infertility!

The AWE Network

The Amazing Women Entrepreneurs Network is a rapidly growing supportive community of tens of thousands of women who are inspired to take their business and life to the next level.

As you begin taking action to create and build your dream life and business, the Amazing Women Entrepreneurs Network is an invaluable resource. It's a place to come for the advice, information, and support that will make your journey efficient and fun.

Here, you'll find all in one place the community, accountability, education, support, exposure, opportunities, resources, and inspiration you need to build a thriving business around your unique gifts!

Visit amazingwomenentrepreneurs.com and discover:

• **Several gifts designed to give you expert advice on building your business**, including tips and strategies for increasing your visibility, creating a profitable, automated sales funnel, working toward financial freedom, slaying Instagram, and so much more (new gifts added often)!

• **A content-rich blog, with posts about every aspect of living your entrepreneurial dream life,** such as how to attract more clients with content you already have, what to look for in a coaching certification, how to develop new blog topics, and more.

• **Online training courses designed to help you grow your business,** using proven, step-by-step processes that will boost your income, help you transition from a 9-to-5 to your entrepreneur dream life, and more.

• **Opportunities to increase your exposure** through our vast network of supportive, positive women entrepreneurs.

• And more.

If you'd like a taste of what the Amazing Women Entrepreneurs Network can do for you, check out all the invaluable gifts at amazingwomenentrepreneurs.com/free-goodies.

The Hope Book Series

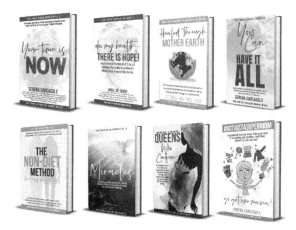

We're on a mission to create a movement of holistic success for women around the world, by sharing real-life stories of people who were able to create lives they love AND businesses that give them the freedom lifestyle they deserve.

That's what the "Hope Book Series" is all about.

It covers topics including business, money, health, spirituality, careers, life, mindset, overcoming trauma, and transformation.

Published books available on Amazon, and more coming soon!

Become a Co-Author of the Hope Book Series

If you want to bring your brand or movement into the world in a BIG Way, then the Hope Book Series is for you!

The Hope Book Series is for anyone looking to bring their products, brand, or service into the world with integrity and power that lights up your life. It's about growing a business you are deeply in love with, making an incredible living *and* impact as you help millions around the globe.

Getting yourself or your brand "omnipresent" is the answer to consistency and profits. Because when it comes to success, it's NOT who you know—it's WHO KNOWS YOU!

We too are on a mission to create a movement of success for women around the world, so they can live a life they love and have a business that provides them the freedom lifestyle they deserve.

The Amazing Women Entrepreneurs Network believes it takes five pillars to THRIVE. Those pillars are Business, Wealth, Mind, Body, and Spirit. When one pillar is broken, it affects the others.

We aim to educate and empower women about taking a holistic approach to enjoying a thriving life.

If you love the "Chicken Soup for the Soul" inspirational books, then you will love our Hope Book Series for women.

Right now, we are accepting co-author applications for upcoming anthologies in the "Hope Book Series." (Topics include business, money, health, spirituality, career, life, mindset, overcoming trauma, transformation, and so on.)

To learn more about becoming a contributor, visit amazing-womenmedia.com.

Hashtag It

Join us in our mission to help women across the globe achieve financial independence and live the life of their dreams by spreading the word!

Every month, I'll randomly choose one person to receive a free gift! If you'd like a chance to win, share a photo of you with this book on social media with the hashtag #HOPEBOOKS.